STRATEGIES AND TECHNIQUES IN FAMILY HEALTH PRACTICE FOR EMPOWERING CHILDREN AND ADOLESCENTS

STRATEGIES AND TECHNIQUES IN FAMILY HEALTH PRACTICE FOR EMPOWERING CHILDREN AND ADOLESCENTS

Edited by

Mary Ann Jennings
John Gunther
Anne B. Summers

Studies in Health and Human Services
Volume 52

The Edwin Mellen Press
Lewiston•Queenston•Lampeter

Library of Congress Cataloging-in-Publication Data

Strategies and techniques in family health practice for empowering children and
  adolescents / edited by Mary Ann Jennings, John Gunther, Anne B. Summers.
      p. cm. -- (Studies in health and human services ; v. 52)
   Includes bibliographical references.
   ISBN 0-7734-6283-X
    1. Family--Health and hygiene. 2. Family social work. 3. Family medicine. 4. Family
therapy. 5. Problem children--Services for. 6. Problem youth--Services for. I. Jennings,
Mary Ann. II. Gunther, John Joseph, 1946- III. Summers, Anne B. IV. Series.

   RA418.5.F3.S774 2005
   616.89'156--dc22

                                                                          2004042325

This is volume 52 in the continuing series
Studies in Health and Human Services
Volume 52 ISBN 0-7734-6283-X
SHHS Series ISBN 0-88946-126-0

A CIP catalog record for this book is available from the British Library

The Edwin Mellen Press   The Edwin Mellen Press
Box 450   Box 67
Lewiston, New York   Queenston, Ontario
USA 14092-0450   CANADA L0S 1L0

The Edwin Mellen Press, Ltd.
Lampeter, Ceredigion, Wales
UNITED KINGDOM SA48 8LT

Printed in the United States of America

This book is dedicated to

Millie Charles
-J.G.

and

Ian Michael Summers
Drake Louis Grimm
Cora Pearl Grimm
Annabelle Rose Eiffert
Josephine Westbrook Eiffert
-A.B.S.

and in memory of

Mary Ruth Jennings
-M.A.J.

TABLE OF CONTENTS

LIST OF ILLUSTRATIONS

PREFACE

Lola M. Butler

Southwest Missouri State University

The family health perspective as conceived in this book is a relatively new phenomenon in the human service field. The message of the family health perspective is ecological and holistic in its pursuit of "family health." This book on family health is a first in that it specifically takes a developmental perspective by looking at the needs of children and adolescents within various contexts. The chapters that follow have an enduring theme of empowerment for families and are premised on the fact that healthy families, in whatever form, are the most important constant in the lives of children and adolescents.

This book represents multiple professional perspectives on family health such as social work, psychology, and nursing and each author shares his or her own extensive practice experience to illuminate the subject matter. The book also provides specific practical practice guidelines for bringing families to health and maintaining them.

Jennings, Gunther, and Summers have made a significant contribution to the development of the family health perspective by the range of diverse chapters they have selected to include in their book. The book does a good job of demonstrating the continued development and maturation of the family health perspective. Finally, this book is an empowering, empathetic statement on children and adolescents and the families that care for them.

Acknowledgements

In completing this book, many have provided encouragement and support, but two persons to whom we are particularly indebted are Kristene Sutliff and Anup Jonathan. Dr. Sutliff, Professor of English, Southwest Missouri State University, put extraordinary time and effort into editing the final draft. We are especially grateful for her frank critiques delivered with such a delightful sense of humor. Mr. Anup Jonathan, a graduate assistant in the School of Social Work at Southwest Missouri State University, exhibited enviable patience and good humor as he used his exquisite word processing skills in completing the tedious job of formatting the final copy.

All the editors owe a special debt of gratitude to all the client families, students and colleagues who have taught us so much about the essential nature and importance of family health and wellness. Of course, we would be remiss if we did not recognize and applaud our immediate and extended families for the living laboratory they provide in which we can be participant-observers in the dynamics of family life. It would be impossible to quantify the ideas, insights, and challenges they have provided that stimulated our quest to achieve a greater understanding of how to help families be healthy so they may provide a healthy headstart for children and adolescents.

Dr. Gunther wishes to acknowledge particularly, Professor Millie M. Charles, Southern University at New Orleans, his lifelong professional mentor and personal friend, for her continuous support and guidance. She has been an invaluable asset in his career as a professional social worker and educator.

Introduction

Work with families has long been a proud tradition in the human services. Much of this work has focused on families with child and adolescent members, as evidenced by the proliferation of public and private sector agencies serving these populations.

Services for children and adolescents historically have taken either an individualistic approach that often exclude or limits the involvement of the family (e.g., in residential treatment facilities) or a family approach framed within the parameters of the family therapy model. In family therapy models the treatment provider works with individuals within the context of the family. For example, in Structural Family Therapy (Minuchin, 1974), the focus is on changing the way in which each part or member of the family system relates to each other and to the family's social context.

With the advent of family-centered practice (Hartman & Laird, 1983), there was a paradigm shift to dealing with family dynamics and interactions instead of focusing on individuals within the family. In this tradition, family health practice (Pardeck & Yuen, 1999) extended Hartman's paradigm to include policy and community considerations as they impact families in an advanced generalist practice context.

However, the family therapy, family-centered and family health perspective lack a focus on practice with children and adolescents, and it is often children and adolescents and their needs and problems that spur families to seek and/ or receive treatment. This book extends the family health perspective, which is described in Chapter 1, to interventions with children, adolescents, and families facing a variety of issues.

In family health practice, the target of change is the family, not the individual within the family. Within an ecosystems framework, a family health practitioner assesses and treats seven domains of family life, i.e., the physical, emotional, mental, spiritual, economic, cultural and social domains. Children and adolescents play active roles in all seven domains of a family's health, yet no book exists that demonstrates how to empower families to meet the needs of and enhance the strengths of their children and adolescents.

In this book, contributing authors describe family health practice in various settings and fields of practice in which they have expertise (e.g., play therapy). The authors address issues and arenas that practitioners often find most difficult (e.g., child protective services, juvenile sexual offenders, and truancy) and present family health approaches to assessing and treating the family holistically.

CHAPTER 1

The Family Health Perspective:
Beyond Family-Centered Practice to Empower Children and Youth

Mary Ann Jennings

Anne B. Summers

Frank G. Kauffman

Corey is 14 years old and has been in trouble with the law since he was 10, when he was caught breaking windows and setting fires in abandoned buildings in his neighborhood. Corey has shoplifted from Wal-Mart and other stores, vandalized school buildings, and broken into neighbors' houses. Most recently, he has been incarcerated for armed robbery. Corey's parents say he has been uncontrollable since he was six years old; he refuses to abide by their rules and has verbally and physically assaulted them on many occasions. Corey is currently expelled from school for beating up another student. The family is at a loss.

Jamie is six years old and has been in and out of a local acute psychiatric facility for the past two years because her behavior is beyond her mother's understanding and control. She has daily rages in which she often hurts her two younger siblings and the family dog. Hospital staff recently diagnosed Jamie with attachment disorder and recommends that she be hospitalized for an extended period of time with regular family therapy. However, there is no long-term psychiatric facility in the area and Jamie's mother must work two jobs to support the family. Jamie's mother is at her "wit's end" about what to do.

Danny is 16 and was born with mental retardation. He attends a local high school and works part-time in a small, locally owned grocery store. Danny is a large young man who recently has become aggressive with his parents and others. He seems to become angry easily and then loses control when he yells and shoves people and things around him. Danny has started disobeying his parents and has talked more about wanting to do what other boys his age get to do. His parents are older (in their early sixties) and are scared for Danny and what will happen to him if he keeps up this behavior. Nothing they have tried with Danny seems to work.

What do these children, adolescents, and families have in common? It depends, in part, on how one views them and their situations. One perspective would see the problems they are experiencing as a disease and trust a professional to "cure" them. Another approach would treat the children and adolescents individually because, after all, they are the ones displaying the problem behavior. A different view would see the inherent strengths of the individual family members, including the children, adolescents, and adults, as well as the family as a whole. The focus would then be on strategies and solutions to enhance the health and functioning of the individuals within the family as well as the family unit.

The focus of this book is family-health-centered social-work practice. This model/paradigm combines various aspects of each of the above perspectives while extending practice to children and families with an emphasis on health promotion emphasizing the cultural, economic, emotional, mental, physical, social, and spiritual needs of the family.

Family-health practice does not deny the existence of problems because that is how children, adolescents, and families identify them. However, family-health practice translates those problems into unmet needs and seeks to remove the blocks that keep individuals and families from meeting their needs. In family health practice, the family is the primary unit of attention, although a practitioner may find occasion to work individually with particular members.

In family health practice, professionals and families identify strengths and build on them to resolve problems together and in doing so promote the healthy functioning of the family. Professionals make a concerted effort to emphasize the medical/pathological model by recognizing and attempting to understand family resilience (Walsh, 1998). An attempt is also made to avoid the bias to perceive healthy functioning with the assumed norms of intact, white, middle-class families and to celebrate diversity with regard to class, ethnicity, sexual orientation, family, and spirituality (Hartman, 1995).

It is the purpose of this chapter to describe family health practice in comparison with more traditional models, its theoretical underpinnings and its usefulness in practice with children, adolescents and families. The book also reflects the emergence of some of the new movements in practice in the last quarter century. Integral to family-health-centered social-work practice, but not necessarily mutually exclusive, are some of the movements identified by Reid (2002) that include the generalist, ecosystems, ecological perspective, strengths perspective, empowerment, task-centered, psychoeducational, solution-focused, multicultural, family preservation, and empirical practice movements.

What Is a Family?

A non-traditional, constructionist conceptualization of the family is used to define and describe family. A family is

> "a system of two or more interacting persons who are related by ties of marriage, birth, or adoption or who have chosen to commit themselves to each other as a unit for the common purpose of promoting the cultural, economic, mental, emotional, physical, social, and spiritual growth and development of each of its members." (Pardeck & Yuen, 1999, p. 1)

This concept of family is chosen because it is the most inclusive and realistic for social/human services workers, their clients, and the community to embrace. Children and adolescents generally have no input into the selection of their families. Their families often do not fit the traditional ideal of happily married mother and father raising healthy and well-adjusted children. So, in order

3

to assess adequately the persons in the family environment, plan interventions that result in positive outcomes, and develop meaningful evaluations, all the significant members of children's and adolescents' families must be recognized and included.

Failure to identify and assess all the members of a family may result in disastrous consequences for children and adolescents. For example, when the parent-like relationships of the parents' potentially abusing girlfriends or boyfriends to children and adolescents are not identified and assessed, the result is often physically and emotionally hurt and damaged children and adolescents. On the other hand, very positive and productive relationships for children and adolescents can be missed when social/human services workers and the community are unwilling to look beyond the boundaries of traditional definitions of the family. A case in point occurs when children and adolescents are denied access to the strengths of healthy and positive gay and lesbian parents on the basis of their sexual orientation.

Children, Adolescents and Families

The numbers of children and adolescents coming to the attention of formal agencies have increased dramatically over the years (Gustavsson and Segal 1994, Kagan and Pritchard 1996, and Boyd-Franklin, 2000). The number of children receiving psychiatric treatment has increased, the number of adolescents receiving psychiatric treatment has grown, and the number of children and adolescents entering foster care has grown exponentially (Knitzer 1996, Littell and Schuerman 1999).

About 30 percent of children in foster care are teenagers (Child Welfare League of America, 1998). Compounding the problem is the fact that approximately 20,000 young adults leave foster care each year with no identified long-term family and no particular place to go (Cook, 1992). With the extension of the period of adolescence well into the 20s in industrialized countries, this is a challenge that very few have been willing or able to address. Children of color continue to be over-represented in foster care: 43 percent are black, 15 percent are Latino, 1 percent are American Indian/Alaska native, and 1 percent are Asian Pacific Islander (Children's Bureau, 2000).

The number of children who are committing criminal offenses has grown and the children ever younger. The number of adolescents convicted of felony offenses and certified to stand trial as adults has also increased. (Hall 1983, Weisheit and Culbertson 1990, Elikann 1999). In addition, federal statistics indicate that substance abuse among adolescents is increasing after achieving relatively lower levels in the early 1990s (Hodge, Cardenas, & Montoya, 2001, p. 153).

Hodge et al. (2001) go on to report that a "growing body of research has indicated that religiosity tends to be a protective factor for substance use by youths (p. 153). Yet, Scott (2003, p. 117) finds that the "significance of spiritual development for the theory and practice of child and youth care professionals and educators has not been extensively explored," and Piechowski (2001) reports that childhood spirituality is almost nonexistent in transpersonal psychology (p. 1). Therefore, professionals who treat substance abusing adolescents are ill-prepared to use this domain of youths' lives to help the teens develop resilience to negative factors occurring in their lives.

Unmet basic physical needs also bring children to the attention of public and private social services agencies. Thirteen million children were food insecure in 2002, of whom 567,000 were considered to be hungry (Children's Defense Fund, 2004). Children "enjoy" the highest poverty level for any group—16.3 percent of children under age 18 lived below the poverty level in 2001 (Joint Center for Poverty Research, 2004).

Explanations for these trends include the demise of the traditional nuclear family and family values, the disintegration of neighborhoods and communities, and an economy that requires two parents to participate in the workplace. These reasons spawn circumstances that cause children, adolescents and families to experience difficulties beyond their control. For example, an economy that embraces fiscal policies that require two parents to work coupled with high cost child care, creates a population of latchkey children before and after school.

5

Research has shown that unsupervised children are often those who commit crimes. (Wright & Cullen 2001 and Martens 1997) The disintegration of close, caring neighborhoods reduces the numbers of adults who supervise and monitor children, thereby leaving children free to make decisions and act in ways that get them into trouble.

Regardless of the causes of the increased difficulties experienced by children, adolescents, and families and the problems they create for the larger society, it is evident that more children and adolescents are experiencing more severe and traumatic events that produce long-lasting consequences for the children and their families as well as for society. For example, child welfare experts maintain that the children entering that system are more damaged than in the past. In addition, children and adolescents are often served by more than one system of care, e.g., mental health, child welfare, juvenile justice with little or no coordination of services.

Traditional Practice with Children and Adolescents

The medical model and traditional developmental knowledge have historically dominated practice with children and adolescents. Practitioners would seek out the cause of the problems experienced and displayed by the children and adolescents and then find a "cure" for those problems. The use of this approach to treating children and adolescents is evident in the numbers of children and adolescents treated in psychiatric facilities and the number of diagnoses based on the DSM IV-TR relating to childhood and adolescent disorders (Johnson, Cohen, & Smailes 2000, Wright et al, 2001).

Just as in the medical profession, human services professionals have traditionally imbued themselves and other professionals with the responsibility and abilities to define and treat childhood and adolescent disorders. The child has been the primary unit of attention of treatment, e.g., when children are placed in juvenile justice or mental health facilities miles from relatives and families.

The involvement of families in their child's treatment is affected by the approach of the professionals and the perspective of the family. Families have often not been included in treatment programs (due to distance and other

6

economic factors such as insurance companies' lack of coverage for family therapy), have been blamed for their children's problems, or have been relieved of involvement because it is easier and less complicated for professionals. Part of the complexity is the perplexing problem for the social/human services worker in defining the child's and adolescent's family. Some children and adolescents have multiple and/or non-traditional families, which makes it difficult to decide who should be included in the intervention strategy. For example, with parents who share joint custody (and both may now have blended families) and share equally the physical custody, does the professional include just the biological parents in the treatment plan or both blended families?

Another barrier for many families is the inaccessibility of professionals' working hours. Time, distance, and money often dictate the treatment decisions rather than the optimal strategies to improve life for the children and adolescents in their families.

If families have been involved in their children's treatment, their inclusion was typically tangential to the treatment process, e.g., keeping family members informed of a child's progress, soliciting information from the families and advising families of what they need to do. Because they are exhausted and confused, families often want to blame or scapegoat the adolescent or child for the problems the family is experiencing. A practitioner following a medical model would allow the family to abdicate its responsibility to and ownership of the problems because the focus was on curing the cause of the problems, i.e., the acting-out child or adolescent. Traditional therapies used with children and adolescents also tend to focus on the individual (e.g., psychodynamic and behavior modification).

Human-services professionals have typically used traditional knowledge in their assessment and treatment of children and adolescents. For example, in treating adolescents, practitioners typically use stage-based developmental theories such as Erickson's Eight Stages of Psychosocial Development. In Erickson's model, the primary task of healthy adolescence is the establishment of an independent identity in order to move into young adulthood. However, there is evidence that adolescence may be about negotiating a new contract of interdependence with parents/caregivers rather than separating from families of origin. (Snyder and Ooms, 1992). Traditional models of development, i.e., psychoanalytical, psychosocial, cognitive, behavioral, and cultural follow individualistic patterns rather than include the social context in which the person is developing.

Family-Centered Practice

In contrast to medical and individual approaches to treatment and in recognition of the person-in-environment perspective central to ecological practice, many professionals have shifted their focus to the family as the primary unit of attention and service (Hartman & Laird, 1983). The orientation of family-centered practice is "toward the family as a major force in adolescent development and the primary resource for most adolescents. The fundamental assumption of family-centered treatment suggests the best way to help a troubled adolescent is to support, strengthen and empower his or her family" (Snyder and Ooms, 1994, p. 3).

In the same vein, an optimal approach to family health centered treatment model for highly vulnerable families is one in which parents and children are encouraged to live together for a lengthy period of time in supervised, structured living arrangements. "These programs also provide comprehensive individualized services to both the parent and child, as well as services to strengthen the family unit and promote family and economic stability" (Allen & Larson, 1998, p. ix). However, a wide variety of treatment programs are needed to serve the multiplicity of needs identified by families and communities.

Family-centered practice, in which the family is the primary unit of attention, is based on family systems theory. Families having difficulties are families experiencing extremes in the concepts of systems theory. For example, families in which children and adolescents have problems may be extremely open and chaotic or extremely closed and secretive. Boundaries between subsystems may be blurred so that children and adolescents assume roles for which they are not prepared. Such extremes cause children to develop ways of coping that are

8

hazardous to their healthy development and that get them into trouble with the larger society. Other systems theory concepts define family-centered practice. For example, families have norms and rules that govern behavior and reinforce or punish such behavior.

When working with families as the unit of service delivery, there are specific principles that guide family-centered practice (McWilliam, Winton & Crais, 1996 p. 2). These include (1) recognizing child and family strengths, (2) responding to family-identified priorities, (3) individualizing service delivery, (4) responding to the changing priorities of families, and (5) supporting family values and lifestyles.

Family-centered practice focuses on the strengths of families and dramatically changes how traditional knowledge is used with children, adolescents, and their families. For example, traditional developmental knowledge focuses on what is wrong with children and adolescents. In family-centered practice, developmental assessment emphasizes what is working for the child and family and identifies, with the family, what they want to work on.

In family-centered practice, children and families move from being clients to being allies and collaborators in the helping process. A family-center approach, as defined by Helflinger and Nixon (1996, p. 25-26) seeks to answer the following questions:

> (a) What are the unique needs of the family members as they define them? (b) What are the strengths (as opposed to deficits) and resources of this family including formal and informal supports? (c) What role do formal services have in addressing the needs of families? (d) What are the preferences of the family with regard to the type, timing and location of services? (e) How can a system be designed that is flexible and responsive to the changing needs of families?

The emphasis should be on the family's definition of needs and on their strengths, preferences, and flexibility.

Family Health Practice

Family-health practice incorporates and builds on the family-centered approach to practice. It relies on a systems or ecological perspective, which understands that a person does not live in a vacuum but instead impacts and is impacted by his/her environment. Part of an individual's environment is her/his family.

In family-health practice the family is the unit of service delivery because of the overwhelming importance of the family unit to developing children and adolescents. As the unit of attention, families actively participate in the helping process and in accordance with the strengths perspective become the directors of the intervention process. The social worker becomes a consultant and collaborator with the family in assessing needs and determining treatment goals.

In a family-health approach problems are translated into unmet needs. The practitioner then looks for what is keeping those needs from being met, which may exist within the family and/or in the family's environment. Identifying needs reduces the stigma of problems that bring with it a stigma that prevents many people from seeking assistance.

However, family-health practice exceeds family-centered practice, which is typically limited by the setting in which the professional operates. Family health is the holistic well-being of the family system and is manifested by the development of and continuous interaction among the physical, mental, emotional, social, economic, cultural, and spiritual dimensions of the family, which results in the holistic well-being of the family and its members (Pardeck & Yuen, 1999). Family health depends on the fullest development possible in each of these domains, and therefore family-health practice is not limited by any particular practice setting.

Another way family-health practice extends family-centered approaches is the manner in which it merges two large areas of theory – family theories (shared with family-centered practice) and health/wellness theories. The family-health practitioner promotes the health of the family in all seven domains. The family-health social worker is not content to simply help a family adapt; the worker helps

10

the family achieve "health" in each area, as defined by the family and as required by external systems (e.g., juvenile court).

Family Health Practice with Children and Adolescents

As can be surmised, family health practice is a new paradigm that utilizes the family as the primary focal system for intervention. This perspective is particularly important in work with adolescents and children, who are dependent on their families for support, guidance, and nurturance.

If there is to be "family health," children and adolescents need the familiarity of the family as a source for networking and support. Additionally, the structural processes imbedded in family interactions (i.e., communication, decision-making, and problem-solving) need to be reinforced so as to empower the child and adolescent. This empowerment process is then extended into the community, and both the internal and external issues that the child and adolescent experience in the family can be resolved. In this process, family health provides a format that allows for the development of children and adolescents through strengthening families.

Book Focus

With this introduction to family health practice with children, adolescents and their families, the remaining chapters of this book describe how the model applies to practice with children and adolescents and their families in various fields and settings. Whatever the field or setting, the goal of all communities and professionals is to provide all children and adolescents with the resources that are associated with positive child development. Schriver (2004) summarizes needed resources as follows:

- adequate nourishment
- good health and access to health services when needed
- dependable attachments or parents or other adult caregivers
- more than one consistently involved adult who provides economic resources, interaction, support, regulation, and positive role modeling to the child
- firm, consistent, flexible discipline strategies

11

- social support and guidance when faced with adversity
- protection from physical and psychological harm
- cognitively stimulating physical and social environments
- play activities and opportunities to explore
- meaningful participation in community life appropriate for age and ability
- access to resources for special needs (p. 39)

Each of the following chapters addresses one or more of the above variables that are associated with positive child development in various settings. By describing its application in these various settings, it becomes evident that the family health practice model can be used effectively with these populations and with a broad array of needs and problems.

References

Allen, M. & Larson, J. (1998). *Healing the whole family: A look at family care programs.* Washington, DC: Children's Defense Fund.

Boyd-Franklin, N. (2000). *Reaching out in family therapy: Home-based, school, and community interventions.* New York: Guilford Press.

Child Welfare League of America. (1998). *State Agency Survey.* Washington, DC: Author.

Children's Defense Fund. (2004). *As national hunger awareness day Approaches, 13 million children face food insecurity.* Press release June 2, 2004. Retrieved June 17, 2004 from http://childrensdefense.org/pressreleases/040602a.asp.

Cook, R. (1992). *A national evaluation of Title IV-E foster care independent living programs for youth, phase 2, final report.* Rockville, MD: Westat, Inc.

Elikann, P. (1999). *Superpredators: The demonization of our children by the law.* New York: Insight Books.

Gustavsson, N., & Segal, E. (1994). *Critical issues in child welfare.* Thousand Oaks, CA: Sage Publications

Hall, J. C. (1983). *Readings in public policy.* National Institute for Juvenile Justice and Delinquency Prevention, Office of Juvenile Justice and Delinquency Prevention.

Hartman, A. (1995). Family therapy. In R. L. Edwards et al. (Eds.) *Encyclopedia of Social Work* (19th ed.) (pp. 983-991). Washington, DC: NASW Press.

Hartman, A. & Laird, J. (1983). *Family-centered social work practice.* New York: The Free Press.

Heflinger, C.R. & Nixon, C.T. (Eds.). (1996). *Families and the mental health system for children and adolescents: Policy, services, and research* Thousand Oaks, CA: Sage Publications.

Hodge, D.R., Cardenas, P. & Montoya, H. (2001). Substance use: Spirituality and religious participation as protective factors among rural youths. *Social Work, 25*(3), 153-161.

Johnson, J., Cohen, P., & Smailes, E. (2000). Adolescent personality disorders associated with violence and criminal behavior during adolescence and early childhood. *American Journal of Psychiatry, 157*(9), pp. 1406-1412.

Joint Center for Poverty Research. (2004). *Poverty information.* (Web site). Joint Center for Poverty Research. Retrieved June 17, 2004 from http://jcpr.org/faq/populations_children.html.

Kagan, S. & Pritchard, E. (1996). Linking services for children and families: Past, legacy, future possibilities. In Zigler, E., Kagan, S. & Hall, N. (Eds.), *Children, families, and government: Preparing for the twenty-first century.* New York: Cambridge University Press.

Littell, J. & Schuerman, J. (1999). Innovations in child welfare: Preventing out-of-home placement of abused and neglected children. In Biegel, D. & Blum, A. (Eds.), *Innovations in practice and service delivery across the lifespan.* New York: Oxford University Press.

Martens, P. (1997). Parental monitoring and deviant behavior among juveniles. *Studies on Crime and Crime Prevention, 6*(2), pp. 224-244.

McWilliams, P. J., Winton, P.J. & Crais, E.R. (1996). *Practical strategies for family-centered early intervention.* San Diego: Singular Publishing Group, Inc.

Pardeck, J. T. & Yuen, F.K.O. (1999). *Family health: A holistic approach to social work practice.* Westport, CT: Auburn House.

Piechowski, M.M. (2001). Childhood spirituality. *The Journal of Transpersonal Psychology, 33*(1), 1-15.

Reid, W. J. (2002). Knowledge for direct social work practice: An analysis of trends. *Social Service Review, 76*(1), 6-33.

Schriver, J. (2004*). Human behavior and the social environment: Shift*ing *paradigms in essential knowledge for social work practice.* 4th Ed. Pearson (Allyn & Bacon): Boston.

Scott, D.G. (2003). Spirituality in child and youth care: Considering spiritual development and "relational consciousness". *Child & Youth Care Forum, 32*(2), 117-131.

Snyder, W. & Ooms, T. (Eds.). (1992). *Empowering families, helping adolescents: Family-centered treatment of adolescents with alcohol, drug abuse, and mental health problems.* Rockville, MD: U.S. Department of Health and Human Services (Substance Abuse and Mental Health Services Administration Center for Substance Abuse Treatment).

Wright, J. & Cullen, F. (2001). Parental efficacy and delinquent behavior: Do control and support matter? *Criminology an Interdisciplinary Journal. 39* (3), 677-706.

CHAPTER 2

When the bough breaks …

Treatment of Children with HIV/AIDS from a Family Health Perspective

Michele Garrison

Nowhere is the importance of utilizing a family-health perspective more clearly illustrated than in the planning of wellness interventions for children living with HIV/AIDS. This chronic and ultimately fatal illness profoundly affects the child and her or his family in all seven domains of family health. In "Chronic Illness and the Family Life Cycle" John S. Rolland discusses how when living with a progressive, incapacitating, and fatal illness (such as HIV/AIDS) the "goodness of fit between the psycho-social demands of the disease and the family style of functioning and resources are prime determinants of successful versus dysfunctional coping and adaptation" (Carter and McGoldrick, Eds., 1999, p. 492).

This chapter will speak specifically about the spiritual, emotional, and social needs for family health, depicted in a composite scenario representing a family living with HIV. Economic needs will be touched on briefly. But before considering this family and family health intervention, a brief review of the history of the epidemic and the state of current medical intervention will be helpful.

Epidemiology and Medical Interventions

The Centers for Disease Control and Prevention (CDC) pinpoints the beginning of the HIV/AIDS epidemic in the United States as 1980-1981. Since that beginning, through the year 2002, the estimated number of children (defined throughout this chapter as under thirteen years of age) diagnosed with AIDS was cumulatively 9,300. In that same time period the estimated number of deaths of children with AIDS was 5,071 (CDC, 2002). In recent years this population has experienced steady declines in the number of AIDS diagnoses and in deaths due to AIDS. This is attributed to encouraging gains in the prevention and treatment of AIDS in three areas affecting children: (a) effective antiretroviral medication protocols available preventively to pregnant HIV- infected mothers (decreasing the number of children born with HIV); (b) earlier diagnosis of at-risk infants (due to accurate testing for infants in the first month of life); and (c) medication protocols now available to HIV-infected neonates, both premature and full-term (The Working Group on Antiretroviral Therapy and Medical Management of HIV-Infected Children [WGA-Child], 2004). Fewer children are being born with HIV, and because of new medication protocols which children can tolerate, more HIV-infected children now have the potential for longer, healthier lives (reaching fuller developmental milestones, both physically and socially) and will progress more slowly to AIDS and death. Research is buying precious time for these young lives and their families until even better medicines and/or a cure is found.

The Family Health Perspective and Children with HIV/AIDS

From the perspective of family health, children and families living with HIV/ AIDS face multiple and progressive challenges that must be addressed in the context of a nurturing environment, which provides for the holistic well-being of the family and each of its members. The family health perspective is a strengths and wellness model. It encompasses not only the problems of and treatments for illness, but also the challenges of living in wellness, and finally the passage into death. Using the strengths and resiliency points of reference, the family health model provides families the means to succeed in all of life's stages. The family health perspective focuses on "prevention, correction, and coping strategies for

16

intractable problems . . . [allowing] the worker to use the strengths of the family and its members to achieve wellness" (Jennings & Skibinski, 1999, p. 46). Though more treatable than ever before, at this time HIV continues to be a
fatal illness. If, however, we view family health, and the health of its members, not only in the context of physical health, but in terms of its " . . . emotional, social, spiritual, and economic well-being our . . . goal is not necessarily to alleviate some deficit but to establish a state of wellness, making the person, persons, or family the best that they can be. It is a self-actualization model for families" (Jennings & Skibinski, 1999, p. 47).

Beyond the increased quality of life and the hope that medical and pharmaceutical progress promises families living with HIV/AIDS, let us look first at some of the unique spiritual, social, and emotional difficulties that challenge these families.

The following case scenario is a composite of several HIV-infected children and their families in the rural U.S. heartland, demonstrating family resources as well as barriers to family well-being:

A Representative Family Study

The Wilson Family:

Residing in an economically depressed rural community of 249
persons; nearest clinic, 60 miles; nearest HIV clinic, 250 miles; nearest pharmacy and grocery, 40 miles; nearest social service agency, 88 miles; no telephone; transportation is an unreliable 1986 car with transmission problems; income between $200.00 and $700.00 per month, depending on family services subsidies and part-time employment for Connie (when available, when she is well enough to work, and when she can barter for child care); family covered by Medicaid; only source of social support is Rick, Connie's on-again, off-again, live-in boyfriend   (whose part time residency could jeopardize welfare benefits).
Mother. Connie Wilson, age 22; single mother; eighth grade education, semi literate; no child support but occasional groceries and car maintenance
contributed by Rickwhen he and Connie are on good terms; HIV positive, infected by husband who died of AIDS five years ago; poor health, CD4-T cell

17

count (the measure of the health of the immune system) declining to AIDS diagnosis.

Children. Jason, age 5; HIV-positive but non-symptomatic with CD-4 count well into normal range; healthy, happy child, completing normal developmental milestones; Jason's father was Connie's former husband who died of AIDS prior to Jason's birth. *Katie,* age 3; HIV-negative; healthy, happy child completing normal developmental milestones; father is mother's boyfriend, Rick.

When we met, Connie and Jason had had a two year history with the HIV/AIDS service agency at which I was newly employed. According to the pediatric treatment protocols of that time, Jason as yet needed no medications for HIV. His care was in a holding pattern of monitoring his normal CD4+ T cell count and caring for the usual childhood maladies. Connie's failing health was the immediate concern.

Blaming the Victim

Judging from clinical notes, the relationship between the agency and the Wilson family had not been a successful one. Connie's file contained only pejorative descriptions of her interactions with the agency. She was characterized as "resistive," "manipulative," "interested only in the subsidies she can get for food, rent and utilities," and most concerning, "a pathological liar." This last referred to her multiple broken promises to keep medical appointments and take prescribed HIV medicines. On the other hand, the record revealed that Connie had scrupulously attended to the children's medical checkups and treatment for minor illnesses. My charge was to make a home visit to see if I could enlist Connie's compliance in her own treatment. It was expected, by the agency, that this effort would fail and that I would close the family's case due to non-compliance. When either Jason or Connie became dangerously ill, it was reasoned, they would be "ready for services," and could re-enter the system. It had been months since an agency case worker had visited this family.

Planning a home visit to the family's remote rural residence was complicated. It was a seven hour round trip drive, mostly on unmarked country roads. Because the roads became impassable when it rained (which it often did), we needed to take into account the long term weather forecasts. Connie could not afford a telephone and her difficulty in reading made it hard to communicate by mail. Nonetheless, after corresponding in very simple language, and with the luck of good weather, we were able to arrange an agreed upon time.

At the time I made a mental note how factors of distance, poverty, and lack of education isolated Connie's family from helping systems. From a person-in-environment perspective, I realized that Connie had worked at least as hard as I had to make this visit possible. That knowledge made me want to understand Connie's "bad-client" behaviors from a different perspective. How should I approach this family to improve their response to health care services? "When intervention does not go well, a practitioner grounded in the disease [rather than the family health] model may blame the client and label ... her as 'non-compliant.' A family health approach ...encourages social workers to [utilize] interactional and reflective process... to become more responsive to the needs of clients and their families" (Pardeck & Yuen, 1999, p. 15). A family health practitioner must pay close attention to client strengths, focusing on systems needs rather than client deficits.

Building Trust and Identifying Strengths

Connie was shy and guarded. Judging by the children's good spirits, cooperative behavior, and the mutual affection between mother and children, Jason and Katie were clearly well cared for. The poverty of their single parent home was another matter. Connie had difficulty finding adequate employment in this depressed rural area. When she did find employment, maintaining regular work attendance in addition to her responsibilities as a mother and homemaker was difficult, because she was so often sick. Connie's CD4+T cell count had been falling indicating that her infection was progressing inexorably to the diagnosis of AIDS and to death. Without the small subsidy she received from family services and the occasional Ryan White grants for rent, food, or utilities, this family would not make it (Federal Ryan White funding includes subsidies for physician visits, hospitalization, medications, medical transportation, food, rent and utilities for eligible indigent and low income persons living with HIV/AIDS.) For child care

19

when Connie could work, and for maintaining her essential car, there was no money: only Connie's ability to barter.

As difficult a client as she had been portrayed, there was something very compelling about Connie. This 22 year old mother loved her children fiercely and was bravely resourceful. She promised that she would keep the medical appointment I would make for her and follow doctor's instructions about taking her antiretrovirals, as long as would help her with this month's staggering heating bill. It had been a brutally cold winter. I was grateful for the opportunity to use utility payment authorization to begin the process of joining with the family.

After this promising start, however, Connie's pattern of going off her medications, getting sicker, and missing medical appointments slowly resumed. I spent the next two years building trust and following up on Connie's falling CD4+ T cell count and medical non-compliance. Jason's CD4+T cell count remained high and he continued to need only regular monitoring. Because I was always able to help her access Ryan White funding for food, rent, and utilities when it was needed, I believed that some brief successes in getting Connie to take her medications was because she was beginning to trust that I cared about her family. But my carrot-and-stick use of the subsides did not resolve her non-compliance no matter how skillfully or creatively I explained the benefits of medication. Watching her health deteriorate, my frustration growing, I caught myself thinking of her in terms of that unproductive and blaming descriptor, "resistant." Connie's excuses, however, for missed physician appointments, and for not being at home for my planned "educational" visits were so painfully inadequate and guilt ridden that my anger over her failing condition, and at being "stood up" after the three and a half hour drive to her home, evaporated in concern and puzzlement. There was a missing piece that eluded me: I was clearly stuck.

In trying to motivate Connie's commitment to self-care, I was not above appealing to her devotion to her children: "What will happen to your children if you die?" The second time I asked her that, we were waiting in the exam room of the only remaining rural physician who would consent to make appointments with her because of the frequency of her "no shows." He was giving us both her last chance. She understood her medical need but could not commit to compliance. "What do I do, Connie, to get you to help yourself?" I threatened, "Do I call children's services to get them to set up permanency planning for your children?" She began to sob, finally risking my understanding.

Depth Assessment and Empowerment

Connie then explained how she had watched Jason's father die a slow, agonizing death in their home from AIDS; his suffering increased, she believed, because of the massive doses of AZT he had been given in those grim days before there were choices and efficacy in medications. She believed that if she took medications that too would happen to her and she would no longer be able to care for her children. She apologized for breaking promises to me, but she had not known what else to do.

Connie, I realized, had made the decision to sacrifice her own health to be able to care for her children. I could not imagine how alone she must have felt, how option-less and desperate. Fighting for the survival of her family, she had used every stratagem at her disposal to feed, clothe, warm, and be with her children. Masterfully and intermittently, she had rewarded my efforts with the rare, kept clinic appointment, submitting to frightening blood tests and exams, with evermore disappointing results, occasionally even taking the HIV medication she so feared, to mollify my concern. She had endured all of this, as well as my cajoling visits, to keep her family afloat and connected to the helping system. Wisely she knew that her family would eventually need all the benefits Ryan White funding offered to persons living with HIV/AIDS. I remembered how Connie had been characterized as "manipulative," and as "a pathological liar," realizing this could have been a textbook case study of client strengths in coping with inadequate and insensitive case management. As a primary intervention, reframing these behaviors to Connie from a strengths perspective let her know I understood and respected her.

This was the beginning of a productive period of collaboration between myself and Connie. With this new level trust, she was able to accept my explanation of improvements in HIV medications and to become medication compliant with few lapses. Her CD4+ T cell rebounded back into the safety range and her health improved, enabling her to work more regularly, easing some of the family's financial stressors.

Family Health Review

In terms of family health, the recognition of this client's strengths addressed family needs in the emotional and spiritual domains of family health. The accurate identification and validation of Connie's strengths (love of and commitment to her children, willingness to sacrifice for them, and the courage and wit to make helping systems work for her family) mitigated her isolation with emotional support, and reinforced her belief in her ability to care for herself and her children. When her behaviors were reframed from the context of "bad client" to behaviors that demonstrated courage, devotion, and protection, Connie's sense of self-worth was strengthened. That self-worth coupled with a positive understanding of the newer and safer medications gave her hope, a fundamental component of physical, emotional, and spiritual resiliency (Griffith & Griffith, 2002, pp. 263 – 268). These resources gave Connie the necessary sense of empowerment for facing her family's next challenges.

Calling in the Specialists

When Jason's CD4+ T cell count began to fall, his pediatrician informed Connie that it was time to start what would be his lifetime of taking antiretroviral medicines. Although her old fears about the harmful side effects of HIV medicine returned, because of her positive experiences with her own antiretroviral medications, Connie was willing to learn about and consider one of the new protocols for children. Only a specialist in pediatric HIV/AIDS would be able to prescribe and follow Jason's treatment: the closest was several hundred miles away, in an HIV/AIDS family clinic. Although frightened of large cities, Connie consented to visit this metropolitan clinic. A family friend volunteered to drive the family the 300 miles to the clinic where I would meet them for Jason's appointment, coming 300 miles from a different part of the state.

The meeting began disastrously, Connie's friend having made a wrong turn as she approached the city. We were an hour late on a very crowded clinic schedule which would end before Jason could be seen and given all the necessary tests. I could tell that Connie was overwhelmed by the size of this crowded clinic. It seemed we had traveled all day for nothing and I was not sure I could convince Connie to make the trip again. Recognizing Connie's limits, the staff made the extra effort to accommodate Jason's tests and physician visit. Connie was put at ease in this new setting. While Jason was being seen, Katie played in the clinic's supervised nursery. For the first time, Connie's and Jason's HIV status did not have to be shrouded in waiting room secrecy. The family was able to meet and interact with other HIV-positive parents and children, as well as their family members. Most importantly, Connie was thoroughly briefed on Jason's prescribed medications, and given a toll-free number she could access from a friend's home if she had any concerns about Jason's health and medication side effects. Because this clinic could provide comprehensive family medical and social service care, we discussed transferring Connie's as well as Jason's care to this clinic for all of their needs. (Their home was no further from this clinic as it was from the agency I represented.) Connie needed to get used to the idea but agreed to make a medical appointment for herself to be seen in one month when Jason would return for his follow up visit. Mileage and gasoline vouchers were given to Connie's friend to cover the cost of transportation.

Connie eventually transferred her own services to this clinic (which for purposes of confidentiality I will refer to as the "Metro Clinic") because, in addition to specialized HIV/AIDS medical services, it met so many of the family's psycho-social needs.

The small semi-rural, HIV/AIDS clinic at which I was employed, and through which I worked with Connie and her family, was in many respects a model of comprehensive case management for persons living with HIV/AIDS. It was not, however, funded at that time to provide comprehensive family health services. Its design was primarily to meet the needs of HIV-positive adults and was only marginally able to serve children and families. While it did an excellent job of linking individual clients to physicians and to many other agencies for non-medical needs, it was not funded to address the complex psycho-social needs of families as systems.

In contrast, the Metro Clinic was funded to serve families holistically. A "one-stop-shop" for families, it offered specialized HIV/AIDS medical treatment for both adults and children within a family systems context. At Metro, Connie and Jason's medical appointments could now be scheduled on the same day in the same building. Case-management meetings could also be scheduled that same day, in the same building, to assess and provide comprehensive psycho-social family needs including: treatment adherence services; mental health services such as psycho-social support to caregivers (parents, extended family, and involved friends), peer-family support, individual and family counseling; case management services to access Ryan White Care Act client subsidies, social service, and community resources; family-wellness services such as respite and recreational events for children and adults; and prevention services. The "one-stop-shop" concept has provided increased resources for Connie and her family, while reducing the number of her appointments to access these resources, relieving the burden on Connie's time away from work, and the wear on her car.

Although the transfer of services to Metro ended my relationship with the family, Connie has reported several years later that she and Jason are both not only alive but thriving. Connie has blossomed in the friendships she has made with staff and especially with other HIV-positive mothers and their families. Jason and Katie (remember Katie, Jason's younger HIV-negative sister?) have been able to attend age appropriate psycho-educational and psychosocial support groups on their "family clinic days." They also attend the play group to meet other children. This allows Connie time for "kid-free" consultations with her own physician and social worker. Two of Connie's closest friends who occasionally come to help with the driving are able to attend the support groups for caregivers. Most importantly, Connie has the information she needs to be "medically compliant" for herself and Jason with medication and physician appointments.

The New Scarlet Letter - Barriers to Spiritual and Social Family Health

In the two to three months before Connie transferred all of her services to Metro Clinic both she and Jason were responding well to their medications. Connie's new found sense of empowerment and hope was such that without discussion she decided to reach out to her community. To gain support, she disclosed the reason for Jason's strict medication dosing times (one of which was during the school day) to his teacher. She also disclosed both her own and Jason's HIV-positive status to her church community. This was terrifying news to both the tiny rural school and church, especially to Jason's Sunday School. Representatives from both institutions immediately contacted her with their concerns that the other children and teachers could "catch it." The Sunday School teacher asked that Jason not attend.

In spiritual and social terms, at the precise moment Connie had reached out to her community for wholeness, she and Jason were met with the threat of expulsion. In a protective response to the stigmatization of her child, Connie's impulse was to pull up stakes, move the family 30 miles to another equally small town and new school, and stop attending church. We discussed the plan's flaws: the move would cost more than Connie could afford; word was bound to spread quickly in this closely knit rural area; and without the family's church community they would be virtually isolated from needed social and spiritual supports.

Identifying Mezzo and Macro Interventions

For the family and child facing life with the diagnosis of HIV, there are complex and intertwined spiritual, emotional, and social issues surrounding this illness. A belief that is deeply and widely held among those of the religious right is that ". . . Acquired Immune Deficiency Syndrome (AIDS) is a form of divine retribution . . . (Le Beau, p. 6, Part II) for the sinful life choices of those, who had they been morally "better" people, making morally "better" choices, would have not gotten infected in the first place.". . . The . . . devil can quickly tempt us to act sinfully (James 1:14-15)." "These sins can involve pornography, fornication, adultery, prostitution homosexuality, and other ungodly sexual practices" (The Christian Broadcasting Network, 2004). In this view, the HIV-positive children of such families are seen as innocent victims. But regardless of being viewed as "morally innocent" these children and their families often suffer exclusion by the spiritual community because of "the sins of the fathers" and because of lack of knowledge about how HIV is actually spread. That lack of knowledge is further confounded by religious taboos surrounding human sexual behavior and drug use, behaviors connected with risk of HIV infection.

A second issue is that this very condition of being "punished for sin," a condition of difference, has the potential to be internalized as a state of taintedness in one's being. This amounts to the inescapable, existential condition of being unworthy of the company of others, of being dangerous to others, and of being spiritually irredeemable in the deepest sense of self, an understanding that can extend to the whole family. This sense is reinforced by behaviors related to the condition of shame, such as secrecy (confidentiality) and the telling of half-truths (being sick at home with a "cold" rather than having medication side-effects). "There is emerging evidence to suggest that patients with HIV who fare better in terms of psychosocial variables like stress, social support, coping, and depression also fare better in terms of disease progression and virologic, immunologic, and clinical status . . . [moreover] these variables are amenable to psychosocial interventions" (Safren, Radomsky, Otto, and Solomon (2002). This makes social work intervention that addresses a family's spiritual and psychosocial needs a central task in promoting family health.

A third and more obvious issue for the child and family living with HIV is that of living with, not dying from, an illness that is ultimately fatal. On what spiritual path does such a child and family walk when they must view the "long range," and the attainment of the social rites of passage such as senior prom, the completion of an education, marriage, children of one's own, and others, as milestones not to be counted or perhaps not even to be thought upon? How does a child and family spiritually live into their entelechy when the "long range," as medical science presently understands, is the foreshortened reality of death?

Interventions targeting the macro issue of "God's punishment," the family's need for social acceptance and support by mezzo level community institutions (such as church and school), and the individual's need to feel existentially worthy of life and of having community can be mutually reinforcing. Additionally, simple to understand information about disease transmission and of simple universal precautions can allay needless fear of social interaction with Persons Living With HIV/AIDS (PLWHA).

For the HIV-positive child one of the most critical issues is of the caregiver's and social support systems' understanding of, and relationship to, the illness itself. Deconstructing the belief that HIV/AIDS is deserved punishment can begin "once a person understands its historical and social contexts. With this shift, new openings often appear for resolving old problems" (Griffith & Griffith, 2002, pp. 151 – 155). What if the caregivers and social support systems can be helped to deconstruct the HIV virus as a teleological instrument of God's punishment, to being simply one of earth's trillions of organisms, which, like ourselves or any other creature on earth, is merely trying to survive? What if HIV were not "the wages of sin" anymore than is the common cold (another virus)? What if we related to those with HIV as we do with friends who have "the flu," taking precautions not to "catch" it but certainly not blaming them, deserting them, or shunning them?

If the family and community can grasp this ecological and spiritual sense of themselves within the nature of the cosmos then their sense of being part of the natural flow of life, and the their sense of spiritual wholeness can be preserved. Deconstructive "reframing" is one of the skills of social work, and a very useful one in a culture in denial of not only death but of regular wear and tear. What if communities, institutions and individuals can be supported in the understanding that illness and even death are parts of the rhythm of life, not a personal punishment or even a personal failure? If caregivers and communities could achieve such an ecological understanding of HIV, then they and the HIV-affected family would not suffer doubly from the illness social separation. The HIV-affected family could be protected from stigma and shame that use isolation and despair to conspire against wholeness of self and resiliency. "Resiliency is the ability to recover from trauma and adapt to change. Family health practice relies

27

on the resilient capacities of families to participate in their own healing process using the [concept of protective factors including]... Environmental protective elements [of] networks of...friends, ministers,...teachers; positive school relationships; church memberships and faith in a higher power; and connections with institutions who foster ties to the larger community...social workers' efforts are directed at enhancing ... protective factors to reduce those that prove to be a risk to clients" (Jennings & Skibinski, p.50).

Family Health Intervention Strategies

From a family health perspective the social worker must carry out interventions at the micro, mezzo, and macro levels of practice. Among the family's strengths was Connie's deep spirituality and conceptualization of a loving rather than punishing God, especially in relation to her children. She had also imparted this belief to her children with nightly prayers and Sunday School participation. At the micro level then, spiritual intervention consisted of fully reinforcing this strength, to "inoculate" her against the judgment of those in her community who saw the family as deserving of punishment (Connie had not married Jason's father).

At the mezzo level, Connie and I discussed the possibility of educational outreach to the church and also to the school to dispel unfounded beliefs and fears about HIV transmission. With Connie's permission, I contacted both the school principal and the minister. They readily accepted my offer to meet with school staff, parents, and church congregation to talk with them about the means of contracting HIV, universal precautions, and to answer any and all questions about HIV and how they could remain "safe" while supporting this family (Connie decided not to attend to give everyone a chance to speak candidly about their concerns).

During this time there was a regional epidemic of Hepatitis Type A, which is far more easily passed from person to person in a school or church setting than the HIV virus. The regional departments of health were widely publicizing universal precautions to quell rates of infection. Using this well-known example of a serious, more familiar illness, more easily "caught" than HIV, helped to "normalize" the concept of protection from any disease including HIV (Carrilio, 1988, p. 255 and Krill, 1988 p. 306).

The outcome of these interventions, and discussing and distributing Department of Health publications, on the safety of universal precautions in social interactions with HIV positive individuals, was immediately helpful in freeing many in the community of unfounded fears of "catching it" so that they could support the family. Others, needing time to digest new information before being fully convinced, were able to observe how their peers were used new knowledge of universal precautions to resume interaction safely with the family. It is important to remember that a frightened community also needs a compassionate response to their fear. Communities need coping skills (i.e., knowledge) if they too are to respond with resiliency to the HIV epidemic.

Most helpful to the church congregation was the macro level intervention of deconstructing the notion of HIV as divine punishment. This process was begun in group discussion, utilizing scripture of their own faith (explicated by the minister) as a point of departure: "And as Jesus passed by, he saw a man which was blind from his birth. And his disciples asked him, saying, Master, who did sin, this man, or his parents, that he was born blind? Jesus answered, Neither hath this man sinned, nor his parents: but that the works of God shall be manifest through him" (St. John 9, 1-3, King James Version). The minister helped to facilitate this discussion and was able to follow up with his parishioners at a later date.

Once Connie and her family could again rely on the support of her church and the children's school, even with the reluctant caution of some, she was able to regain a sense of belonging, of connectedness that she could then impart to her children. This sense of wholeness was deeply healing at the spiritual, social, and emotional levels for this family. The alternative of banishment has been from ancient times the most unbearable of spiritual and social sanctions (Aristotle; Qur'an, 059.002; Ezra 7:26, King James Version). Connie had known this intuitively when she had risked the truth of her family's medical problems at church and at school. This family and this community are to be credited with their

29

courage to learn and grow in the face of fear and taboo. The work that Connie did with Jason's school and with their church to keep those systems as supports in their lives, was more than a spiritual and social victory. It was also intrinsic to the success of their medical treatment.

Economic Family Health Needs

While Connie and Jason have responded extremely well to the new and powerful medicines, this by no means typifies the experience of every Person Living With HIV/AIDS (PLWHA). One of the elements critical to the health and survival of patients taking HIV medicines is that of adherence. Lack of adherence decreases pharmaceutical efficacy and can allow the virus to mutate, becoming immune to medicine. This outcome in turn presents a progressively difficult problem for physicians. First of all, there are a limited number of pharmaceutical choices and combinations in treating HIV. Second, not all patients respond well to or tolerate all options. Finding the most effective antiretroviral for a patient can be a difficult task. Once this has been decided upon, patients still must adjust to, or live with, varying degrees of distress often caused by side effects. Some must make the choice between living longer (adherence and living with severe side effects) and quality of life (no medicine, no side effects, shorter life span). There are also the complicated logistics of multiple daily doses that need to be coordinated with food intake. Some medicines must be taken in certain time frames before or after the ingestion of food. Others must be taken with the ingestion of food. Some medicines need refrigeration. And some of the medicines just "taste terrible." Adherence can interfere with or at the minimum complicate everyday activities such as work, school, and recreation (Safren. Radomsky, Otto, and Salomon, 2002). Finally, just because a PLWHA has increased feelings of wellness due to medication effectiveness does not ensure that he or she has enough reserve to return to work and stay well. As chronic survivors, PLWHA, especially children, remain medically fragile. While adherence problems are difficult enough for adults, they can be especially so for children.

To address the issues surrounding medication adherence, intensive psycho-educational and psychosocial support must be in place for the family as a whole as well as involved friends and family outside the home, especially during the early stages of treatment. Care providers must offer these supports to ensure the family's best response to treatment and best hope for wellness and survival. Connie's new Metro milieu more than met these critical needs for her, her children, and support system, especially in view of her original fears about HIV medicines.

One of the important supports that Metro Clinic has provided Connie is a grief group for survivors. She has been able to grieve openly her loss of Jason's father, gaining a sense of dignity for her memories of him and for their relationship. Jason has also been supported in an age appropriate way to talk about his father, his loss, and how he can memorialize him. Katie has formed supportive friendships with other HIV-negative but affected children who understand her fears. Gone is the sense of shame and secrecy. Gone is the isolation of having no one who understands. The special needs of this family are shared and normalized by others living in the same daily circumstances. This in turn empowers the family to carry their sense of wellness back into their small communities, strengthening their local social supports.

Conclusion

In exploring the needs of "The Wilson Family," the complex interaction between multiple domains of family health has been demonstrated. The successes this fictionalized family experienced were due to the optimal meeting of family health needs.

A primary difference in the family's first agency and the "Metro Clinic" is not in an understanding of necessary standards and provisions of care but in funding. The multiple and comprehensive services that were able to address all of this one family's barriers to wellness are expensive but are clearly necessary to holistic family health.

At the macro level of practice, there are two ominous factors in the provision of HIV/AIDS care for children and families. The first is that the number of persons living with AIDS has steadily been rising since 1993, due to the effectiveness of the new medications to keep PLWHA's alive longer. The second ominous fact is that this is also a reflection of the increased rates of HIV infection and AIDS cases. Unfortunately "the Bush Administration's proposed Fiscal Year (FY) 2005 budget has flat-funded virtually all HIV/AIDS care, prevention, and housing programs despite ongoing increases in HIV infections and AIDS cases in the United States. For four years running, the Administration has flat-funded virtually all domestic HIV/AIDS programs. The lone increase proposed for the Ryan White CARE Act is a $35 million boost for the AIDS Drug Assistance Program . . . Unfortunately, this meager increase is nearly $300 million less than California and other states need to avoid joining 15 other states that already have waiting lists, dangerous enrollment caps and other cutbacks in [mediation] access for people with HIV/AIDS" (San Francisco AIDS Foundation, 2004).

When the number of PLWHA's needing medication, basic survival subsidies, psycho-social support, and other essential family health services exceeds the flat line of funding for the Ryan White CARE Act is when the "cradle will fall" in terms of the safety net for children and families.

References

Aristotle, A treatise on government, (Book IV: Chapter XIV)

Rolland , J. S., (1999) Chronic illness and the family life cycle. In Carter, B., and
      McGoldrick, M., (Eds.), The expanded family life cycle: Individual,
      family and social perspective (p. 492). Boston: Allyn and Bacon.

Centers for Disease Control and Prevention. HIV/AIDS Surveillance Report
      2002; 14: (Tables 3 & 7). Retrieved February 1, 2004 from
      http://CDC.gov.pdf

Carrilio, T. E., (1988). The psychosocial rehabilitation model: An ideology of
      social functioning. In R. A. Dorfman (Ed.), Paradigms of clinical social
      work (p. 255). New York: Brunner/Mazel Publishers.

Griffith, J. L., & Griffith, M. E., (2002). Encountering the sacred in
      psychotherapy (pp. 151 – 155 and pp. 263 – 268). New York: The
      Guilford Press.

Krill, D. F., (1988). Existential social work. In R. A. Dorfman (Ed.), Paradigms
      of clinical social work (p. 306). New York: Brunner/Mazel Publishers.

Jennings, M.A. & Skibinski, G. J. (1999). Treating families through the family
health perspective. In J. T. Pardeck & F. K. O. Yuen (Eds.), Family health:
A holistic approach to social work practice (pp. 46-53). Westport,
Connecticut: Auburn House.

Le Beau, B.F. (n.d.) The political mobilization of the new Christian right (p. 6,
Part II). Retrieved February 10, 2004, from http://are.as.wvu.edu

Pardeck, J. T., & Yuen, F. K. O., (1999) A family health approach to social work
practice. In J. T. Pardeck & F. K. O. Yuen (Eds.), Family health: A
holistic approach to social work practice (p. 15). Westport, Connecticut:
Auburn House.

Safron, S. A., Rodomsky, A. S., Otto, M.W., Salomon E. (2002). Predictors of
psychological well-being in a diverse sample of HIV-positive patients
receiving highly active antiretroviral therapy. Psychosomatics, *43*(6), 483.

San Francisco AIDS Foundation Newsletter (February 3, 2004). Retrieved
February 24, 2004 from http://www.sfaf.newsroom.fy05_budget

The Christian Broadcasting Network (2004). Keys to powerful living:
Overcoming sexual sin (p. 2). Retrieved February 22, 2004, from
http://www.com/spirituallife/cbnteachingsheetskeys
overcoming_sexual_sins.asp

The Working Group on Antiretroviral Therapy and Medical Management of HIV-
Infected Children (2004). Guidelines for the use of antiretroviral agents in
Pediatric HIV-infected children (pp. 15 – 16). National Resource Center at
the Francois-Xavier Bagnoud Center, UMDNJ. Retrieved February 1,
2004 from http://AIDSinfo.gov.pdf

Chapter 3
Truancy: Engaging the Family
Regina Goff

Scotty wakes up mid-morning and warily looks at his bedside clock. He quickly decides that he probably will not attend school today unless his mother forces him to get out of bed and get dressed. Experience assures him that she likely will not. Besides, the family was awake until very late last night watching a video. Scotty also remembers he has a science test today but is keenly aware of being so far behind in his homework that he is unfamiliar with the concepts or terms likely included in this test. Actually, he feels a bit overwhelmed thinking about all his missing assignments. Oh well, he will just go back to sleep. After all, Scotty's mother has mentioned repeatedly that having a high school diploma is overrated. No one in Scotty's family earned a high school diploma, and they appear to be making their way, so why should he worry? He turns over and goes back to sleep.

Given the estimates that "47 million Americans cannot read or write at all," and "75% of prison inmates in the United States are illiterate," the obvious intent to encourage each American child to earn a high school diploma is for the good of the child as well as the larger society (American Bar Association, 1987). Research shows that earning power in adulthood is directly correlated to educational attainment. Cantelon and LeBouef (1997) advise that dropouts who are employed full time have a median income half that of high school graduates. These pragmatic factors coupled with a concern for marginalized children and families should encourage social workers to focus practice attention on truant students and their families.

Definition of Truancy

Truancy is typically and simply defined as when a school-aged child refuses to attend school. While truancy can occur at any age and be provoked by myriad factors, this discussion will focus on students who are approximately eleven years old and older. Truant students may be absent from school one day per week or may attend school only one day per week.

Most states have enacted legal statutes that require children to be in regular school attendance and place that burden on parents. States' requirements are similar regarding age and education intent of school-aged children, and in most states a child's parents or guardians are held responsible for their child's school attendance and may face legal repercussions (Department of Education, 2001) if found guilty of not ensuring regular school attendance. Parents or guardians may face monetary fines or in severe cases, incarceration. Given these guidelines and demands, the student's family must be the focus of social work holistic intervention.

Definition of Educational Neglect

In contrast to the child who refuses to follow a parent's instruction to attend school, educational neglect occurs when parents do not ensure their children regularly attend school. The reasons for and causes of educational neglect are as varied and unique as each family. Socioeconomic status, family makeup, family mobility, family pathologies, death in the family or even divorce can greatly impact a student's school-attendance rate. Perhaps more importantly the immediate family structure and functioning are very powerful and influential to a child within that family.

Parents who do not make school attendance a priority may face legal prosecution for educational neglect. If families find themselves in this position, they may be forced to address underlying issues including substance abuse, homelessness, and domestic violence, which clearly contribute to truancy. For some families, law enforcement involvement may force immediate interventions focusing on truancy as well as other familial pathologies that otherwise may be not be addressed.

Family Perspectives of Truancy

Families of frequently truant students experience truancy differently than students of the general public, often listing reasons to allow or seemingly encourage truancy. Family roles, family values, and negative school experiences are among the explanations and situations of truant students' parents.

Most parents and students view daily school attendance as an unwritten rule of acceptable behavior. Hence, the majority of public school students attend school more than ninety percent of prescribed hours and do not regularly and actively attempt to avoid school. Only a small number of students can be categorized as truant. In the family of a truant child, family roles and family rules may be contrary to the acceptable norms of the larger society, and interventions by social workers will require close observation, preferably within the home environment, along with an understanding that each family is unique and powerful.

As is well documented by Payne's text, *The Framework of Understanding Poverty* (2001), parents of what she terms the "poverty-class" may not be interested in educational attainment and in fact may not see the value of a high school diploma or other educational training. Parents involved in long-term poverty may view high school diplomas as a luxury, not a necessity for success in their world view. Parents may also be fearful of their children's achieving more education than they, which may lead to the children's leaving the neighborhood or having less future contact with the parent and family.

Remaining mindful of Dr. Payne's approach when working with families of truant students will offer insight and tools with which to work. This view allows social workers to be more understanding of many students' and families' values and beliefs and will hopefully lessen practitioner's frustrations. Dr. Payne's interventions include instructing children in the hidden rules of the middle class and acknowledging family values and beliefs while attempting to impact the children's beliefs. Empowering students to take control of their futures through education is the focus of Dr. Payne's work.

Truancy or educational neglect affect and are affected by the family holistically. A child's poor school attendance may occur when the family is struggling with other issues and pathologies. Family members may suffer from substance abuse, mental illness, or other problems. Obviously, if parents or guardians are focused on struggling with the issues and difficulties associated with substance abuse, their child's school attendance may not be of particular importance.

Many family members of truant children have conventional and gainful employment. Parents' work schedules may not allow them to be at home with the children before school, which can place great responsibility on the children to attend to their education. Often unsupervised students are conscientious enough to get themselves to school on a regular basis, and this discipline and drive may facilitate success in academics and in later adulthood.

Underlying Truancy Characteristics

Truancy has many facets and contributing factors. As previously mentioned, the most significant factors relating to school truancy are socioeconomic status, family structure and makeup, family mobility, family pathologies, an external locus of control, educational success and experience of the child and family and school bullying.

School truancy appears to occur more frequently within the lower socioeconomic statuses and especially among students who are marginalized socially and academically. Students of poorer families may feel the pressure of not having acceptable clothing or other material items many of their classmates enjoy. These students may have an unclean odor, often have less strict hygiene regimes than others in their class, and may be forced to wear unclean clothing. Students are known to maltreat others who lack cleanliness. In some families, funds required to launder clothing or to purchase basic hygiene products just do not exist. Whatever the circumstance, bodily and clothing cleanliness should be of particular focus for the social worker working with the family.

Family structure, which for these purposes includes family-member identity, member roles, communication patterns, and intra-family relationships, are crucial to the family's abilities to function. Determining which adult family member is responsible for the children's school attendance is equal in importance to other major household responsibilities and is largely determined through communication patterns and family members' responses. A more effectively functioning family will share and overlap these responsibilities, which in turn will ensure the children attend school. If no adult in the family appears to accept responsibility for the children, school attendance may suffer.

Mobility is a strong contributor to truancy. Students whose household relocates often may not have the opportunity to initiate friendships or become involved in extracurricular activities that encourage school attendance. In addition, teachers may not be able to adjust classroom coursework or provide required tutoring to ensure students are prepared to compete academically when those students may only be in the classroom for a short while.

For most teens, established household routines or schedules that include required school attendance will encourage students to attend school regularly. Routines appear to lessen family chaos and allow students to expect daily school attendance which in turn may avoid fewer conflicts each morning before school.

Consistently truant students frequently explain the reasons for their absences as an external locus of control. An alarm clock not working as expected, or suffering from an ongoing illness, such as asthma, or an automobile that did not start are common reasons for absences or tardiness. Often social workers must inquire thoroughly to determine if illnesses have been formally diagnosed and are actively being treated. In addition, questions must be asked of families regarding financial difficulties to ensure ongoing issues are being addressed. This lack of personal control and responsibility are typically indicative of other underlying issues such as substance abuse, underemployment, or mental health concerns including depression, which will be imperative to address during interventions.

Students who tend to be truant are often students who have experienced significant negative reinforcement by school teachers and administration. In addition, these teens have likely been unsuccessful academically or socially and typically are not involved in extracurricular activities. In short, typically truant students are socially marginalized and do not feel comfortable at school; therefore, they have little motivation to attend daily, much like anyone avoids uncomfortable places (Baker, 2001).

Often students and families complain about bullying by other students while at school. Bullying may explain why parents apparently allow truancy or why children are truant. Bullying can occur at various times during the day, before class, after class and often during class (Baker, 2001). Students are especially vulnerable to bullying at free times, including recesses and lunch times. Bullies do not have to be physically larger than their victims; they rely on the perception by other students that they should be feared.

Effects of Truancy on the Student

Through truancy, many areas of a child's life are affected, especially when poor school attendance begins in the child's early school years. In terms of academics, a truant student is likely to suffer from delayed abilities to read as well as have mathematic abilities at a lower level than their peers. When students' abilities are less than their peers, they will feel inferior and embarrassed in the classroom and truancy can only add to lowering those abilities. Clearly, if children feel unsuccessful in school, they may want to avoid school altogether.

Students who consistently attend school typically participate with various groups or clubs, whether those groups are athletic teams, academic teams or part of an informal group of students. Students may begin to identify with the "smart kids" in a particular class or perhaps the children who choose to confront teachers and administration. Children who do not identify with a student group may feel marginalized. Children who are lost in the crowd, or feel they do not have a specific place, may not feel welcome or even comfortable at school. For those students, staying at home may be preferable even if that means feigning illness or injury.

Academic Implications

Obviously, when students do not attend classes on a regular basis, remaining current academically is all but impossible. Only the most intellectually gifted truant student will not fall dramatically behind his or her classmates academically. Often truant students will have several missing assignments and be woefully behind their peers in academic theories or concepts. Being so far behind their peers academically will only serve to make students feel more uncomfortable, more inept, and further marginalized.

Often children's teachers may not be able or available to offer additional services to allow the child to compensate academically for missing work. Students may require specific and extensive services including academic tutoring and other one-on-one assistance. The most important ingredient for children to compensate for missed work is the students' honest effort and desire to work hard and learn the necessary information. In any case, students will likely require encouragement and positive reinforcement as they undertake this quite daunting task. Even moderately truant children may fall severely behind in assignments and other school work.

Parent Resources

Often, despite a parent or guardian's best and most diligent efforts, a child just will not attend classes. Frustrated parents regularly request services from their school or perhaps from local juvenile justice offices to aid their efforts toward child school attendance. Often parents have been warned by local law enforcement agencies they will be held responsible if their child continues to be truant from school. They may become frustrated and irritated and feel powerless to ensure their child's attendance, but the child continues to refuse to attend school.

Parents may be able to receive assistance from local law enforcement agencies if the family is willing and able to request and then accept agency services with the admission they have little or no control over the child. Obviously, this may be a difficult decision and act for a parent. Parents may be fearful that this indication of their inability to control their child may lead to losing physical custody of their child to their state's family services agency. Conversely, parents may become so frustrated with their children's truancy that they seek help and reinforcement from those agencies.

Consequences of Truancy for the Student

Students are often given consequences for truancy, which may range from a stern lecture by school officials to prosecution by a juvenile justice system. While it is generally acknowledged that school truancy is a precursor to more serious law offenses (Cantelon & LeBouef, 1997), many juvenile justice agencies do not have adequate personnel or facilities to appropriately address truant juveniles. These agencies have discovered that if juveniles are threatened with consequences that cannot ultimately be administered, the corrective effect of that threat is greatly diminished. Hence, in this writer's opinion, many juvenile justice agencies are reluctant to deal harshly with truant juveniles.

By contrast, if a child is manipulated to attend class by threats of punishment or other disciplinary measures, that child may choose to be a behavioral problem in the classroom. Teachers may be asked to contend with a disruptive or disrespectful student who clearly does not want to be there. Students are often savvy enough not to fear or perhaps desire to be placed in a disciplinary setting where they can be in more control of their daily schedule or at least not attend regular classes. In short, suspension may be preferred to attendance in the student's regular classroom.

Motivating Students

Motivating students to attend and excel in academics can be very difficult. If children do not have the appropriate motivation to attend school and actively participate as students, they cannot be realistically forced to do so. Many academic activities demand students actively involve themselves within the classroom setting; however, students cannot be forced to participate. Students may be rewarded for compliant behavior, but it is difficult at best to force children to become students.

Forcing a child to attend school while not impacting his/her motivation to participate appropriately as a student will not ensure an education; it will only impact attendance, until the student is legally old enough to drop out of school. Intrinsic motivation must be cultivated for an individual to excel, engage, or minimally succeed as a student. This motivation may be discovered if social workers recognize the importance of family and attempt to enlist them in the efforts to increase the student's resolve to do well in school.

Practice implications

If the social worker's goal is to forge a strong and *working* relationship with a truant child's family, focusing his/her practice methods with a family-health, strengths perspective is crucial. This approach will enable practitioners to build a proactive base to address problematic behaviors and family pathologies as they appear. The family–health-practice approach encourages appreciation of the "holistic well-being" and uniqueness of each family, which allows the social worker to focus his/her interventions on family interactions and family patterns (Pardeck & Yuen, 1999).

Observance of Maslow's Hierarchy of Needs (Saleebey, 1992) offers a context to view and evaluate the needs of truant children and their families. As is widely recognized, if children's basic needs are not met, a lecture from a teacher or another school administrator, or even formal discipline referral regarding truancy will not be significant. In addition, when a child does not have an adequate, quiet space in the family home to afford the required amount of sleep, or has inadequate nutrition, a small matter like a stern lecture will not impact him/her. As with all of us, if our basic needs are not being met, issues such as education and the like are just not important. As was previously mentioned, home visits will offer great insight and coupled with additional information from other resources will help determine whether that family's basic needs are being met.

If a practitioner discovers that a family is facing homelessness, or the family is suffering from domestic violence or has little money for clothing or food, these issues will obviously need to be addressed before school truancy can be successfully approached. Social workers may need to spend time building rapport and trust before families are comfortable divulging such personal information. After those issues are discovered, investigated, and, if appropriate, a resolution reached, school attendance can be improved as well as the overall family functioning.

When a strengths perspective-practice approach is used, the focus includes viewing the family from the systems theory standpoint. This theory recognizes that a family "can be viewed as a whole made up of individual parts," and interventions should address the family as a whole (Pardeck & Yuen, 1999). To acknowledge what is working well within that family structure and to expand and build upon those behaviors will allow the family to feel empowered and able to successfully overcome their problems (Pardeck & Yuen, 1999). It is always possible to discover positive and functional behaviors within any family. Even the most apparently dysfunctional family may care deeply about each other, be willing to protect each other, and be very close emotionally.

Perhaps the most important aspect of a social worker's practice with families of truant students is advocacy. Advocacy within the school setting, advocacy when working with law enforcement agencies, as well as occasional advocacy on the student's behalf within the family will be crucial to successful practice intervention. Truant students have frequently forged a combative relationship with their teachers and school administrators. If a student chooses to work toward changing his/her behavior, the practitioner may need to intervene with teachers and administrators to encourage a more cooperative relationship. Perseverance will be key for both the practitioner and the student.

In this writer's opinion, parents of truant children often have ineffective parenting skills. Perhaps parents have disciplined their children sporadically or have administered punishment sporadically. Truant students rely on the inconsistency of their parents to allow irregular school attendance. Practitioners must quickly assess the parenting abilities and styles of their clients to determine if parenting classes or similar interventions are required.

Frequently, parents of truant children were not successful in school themselves (Baker, 2001). Most parents of truant children did not graduate from high school and most did not earn high-school equivalency diplomas. Parents are often not comfortable visiting schools or conferring with school administrators or

44

teachers; this discomfort must be addressed and hopefully eased. Social workers may accompany parents during conferences and actively advocate for clients. Modeling positive behaviors will help parents better understand how to interact with school officials.

Many families involved in continual school truancy have also previously experienced intervention by school officials, local law enforcement agencies, or family-service governmental agencies. These families will likely be suspicious and mistrustful of governmental agencies and school administrators especially regarding their children. Social workers working with families of truant students can overcome those prejudices with perseverance and honesty in order to build trust with family members. To be successful with these clients, practitioners must be prepared and willing to advocate for the child and family at their school. In addition, reminding parents of their responsibilities toward school attendance can be difficult but is crucial to impacting the child's attendance.

In this writer's opinion, observing the family within their environment is crucial to understanding the home atmosphere, family roles, family priorities, family member's interactions and family rules. Only then can practitioners discover what the family experiences specifically regarding roles of each family member, family rules, communication patterns, family interactions, and monetary priorities. Because it has been clearly established that truancy is a symptom of other family troubles (Baker, 2001), home visits are crucial to holistic interventions. Only after having a clear overall view of the student's family will practitioners have the knowledge to discover underlying issues and difficulties to address in order to impact school attendance.

Conclusion

As previously stated, truancy is not a pathology occurring in a vacuum. Social workers must be prepared to address not only the student's behavior, but to focus empowering interventions on the family. Being conscientious in terms of the role as diligent family advocate, confronting when necessary and being fully committed to intervene in whatever way necessary will encourage successful practitioner intervention.

The difficult and harsh reality of school truancy is that the student must and will make a choice. S/he may attend school regularly and attempt to do well or may never attend school willingly. The child may choose to become a student; however, social workers would do well to accept that children or teens are clearly in control of this aspect of their lives and are members of a family unit who will develop and adopt their own views regarding school attendance. For this reason and others, a family health focus using a strengths perspective practice methods are effective when working with truant students and their families.

Remaining mindful that truancy is not an isolated pathology within a family, and that many others have attempted to make children attend school will help practitioners focus interventions holistically and proactively. Obviously, addressing family difficulties before they become pathologies will allow the family to avoid problems and the need for intervention. When social workers take the time to discover the family's underlying issues and address them, improvement in truancy will likely follow as will improved family function.

Scotty

Scotty decides not to go to school. He is still in bed sleeping when school officials knock at his door. His mother answers, and Scotty hears her say that she doesn't know why Scotty is still at home. Scotty's mother comes into his room and shakes him awake. After a heated argument, Scotty grudgingly gets dressed and goes to school with the school officials. He is hungry and tired, but lunchtime is just an hour away, so Scotty feels he can wait that long. Scotty indolently mentions that he has a science test today, but realizes he has no realistic hope of making a passing score.

When they arrive at Scotty's school, the school social worker greets them and begins talking with Scotty about his attendance. The social worker gathers information from Scotty and others at the school and begins researching possible resources for Scotty and his family. After a lengthy home visit, she arranges school tutoring for Scotty and parenting classes for Scotty's mother along with intensive in-home counseling. Scotty's mother and the social worker visit his school and speak with Scotty's teachers and the administration about his grades and attendance. Compromises are reached and a plan is developed for Scotty to make up the majority of his missing assignments. Other problems and resources are discussed. The social worker along with Scotty's mother agrees to pursue additional resources to help the family with better housing and a more stable income.

Eventually, Scotty's situation improves and he passes the eighth grade. Scotty stays in school and as a result dramatically decreases his chances of incarceration, of unemployment and of fathering a child out of wedlock; and he increases his future earning potential by one half (Cantelon & LeBoeuf, 1997).

References

American Bar Association, (2001) *Truancy, literacy and the courts.* Standing Committee on Substance Abuse. Retrieved July 25, 2004, from www.abanet.org/subabuse/truancy_brochure.pdf.

Baker, M. L., Sigmon, N., Nugent, M. (2001). *Truancy reduction: Keeping students in school.* Retrieved July 25, 2004, from http://www.ncjrs.org/pdffiles1/ojjdp/188947.pdf.

Cantelon, S., & LeBoeuf, D. (1997). *Keeping young people in school: Community programs that work.* Retrieved July 25, 2004, from http://www.ncjrs.org/txtfiles/dropout.txt.

Curtis, J., & Harris, O. (1997). *Family treatment in social work practice.* Itasca, IL: F. E. Peacock Publishers, Inc.

Day, J. C., & Newburger, E. (2002). *The big payoff: Educational attainment and synthetic estimates of work-life earnings.* Retrieved July 25, 2004, from http://www.census.gov/prod/2002pubs/p23:210.pdf.

Garry, E. (1996). *Truancy: First step to a lifetime of problems.* Retrieved July 25, 2004, from http://www.ncjrs.org/txtfiles/truncy.txt.

Pardeck, J. T., & Yuen, F. K. O. (1999). *Family health: A holistic approach to social work practice.* Westport, CT: Auburn House.

Payne, R., (2001). *A framework for understanding poverty.* Highlands, TX: aha! rocess, Inc.

Saleebey, D., (1992). *The strengths perspective in social work practice.* White Plains, N.Y.: Longman Publishing Group.

National Center for Educational Statistics, (2001). *Digest of educational statistics tables and figures.* Retrieved July 25, 2004, from http://nces.ed.gov/programs/digest/d01/.

Chapter 4

Ethical Implications of Adolescent Suicide

from a Family Health Perspective

Joan E. Goldberg

Anne B. Summers

The suicide of a child or adolescent is a tragic experience that no one can fathom and few people talk about. In its aftermath, family and friends are left with an unimaginable sense of grief and often guilt that never leaves. In this country alone, between the years 1980 and 1992, the suicide rate in children age 10-14 increased 120% (Jamison,1999) with 5000 young people successfully committing suicide per year (Marcus, 1996). These rates may be even higher given that deaths are sometimes misclassified through error and bias (Mohler & Earls, 2001). About one million adolescents out of 25 million attempt suicide each year from which about 276,000 sustain injuries serious enough to require medical treatment (Stone, 2001). Suicide among adolescents 15 to 24 years of age is the third major killer after homicide and accidents (NIMH, 2003). Adolescent boys in the 15 to 19 year range commit suicide at a rate nearly five times as high as the rate for girls (Gould & Kramer, 2001; Allison et al., 2001). A homosexual orientation appears to be a risk factor for suicidal behavior irrespective of gender, or racial or ethnic identity (Barowsky et al, 2001; Garofolo et al., 1999). Among various racial groups the American Indian and Alaskan native have the highest adolescent suicide rates (MacGowan, 2003). Suicide is the second leading cause of death among Caucasian adolescents; among African American adolescents, it is the third leading cause of death (Eckert et al., 2003).

Given these sobering statistics, this chapter will explore the issue of suicide among adolescents within the context of family health practice and the ethical issues health care professionals face when working with young people who are at risk.

Although research has demonstrated an array of risk factors that can be linked to adolescent suicidal behavior, predicting a suicide attempt in an adolescent is an inexact science. Because prediction remains so elusive, social workers must exercise both the art and science of family health social work practice in working with suicidal adolescents and their families. The science is the knowledge and recognition of all the risk factors associated with adolescent suicide attempters and completers. The art is going beyond the traditional approach of concentrating only on individualistic factors to scrutinize closely the interactional dynamics among the seven domains of family health social work practice: cultural, economic, emotional, mental, physical, social and spiritual. (Ayyash-Abdo, 2002; Pardeck & Yuen, 1997).

The Family Health Perspective

Because of the very individual nature of suicide, traditionally it has been studied primarily within the context of individual pathology with only tangential attention focused on family and community. Yet when the literature on risk factors for adolescent suicide is reviewed, it becomes abundantly clear that the risk factors are inextricably associated with the family. For example, risk factors include substance abuse, mood disorders, interpersonal or conduct disorders, prior suicide attempts, and a strong family history of suicide, all of which must be addressed with the entire family for successful intervention to occur (Pelkonen & Marttuven, 2003; Rowan, 2001; Egeland & Sussex, 1985). The family must be assessed from a perspective that empowers the family to identify and build on its strengths in order to develop resilience to pressures (Early & GlenMaye, 2000). Jennings and Skibinski (1999) describe the family health perspective in a way that makes it a perfect fit for working with adolescents with suicidal behaviors: "Family health is a perspective that encompasses prevention, correction, and coping strategies for intractable problems and allows the worker to use the strengths of the family and its members to achieve wellness" (p. 46). Such a perspective is essential to good social work practice with adolescents because the entire family must be healthy to prevent and remediate suicidal behaviors.

Adolescent Suicide

Adolescence is a life stage that is characterized by change and, some believe, turmoil for the child but oftentimes for the entire family. Erikson (1968) noted that the life stage of adolescence is characterized by the psychosocial crisis of identity and identity confusion where the development of identity depends on both inner supports and social supports. The young person works at being an independent self with its own identity. "The failure to resolve developmental crises, as described by Erikson, can lead to the belief that suicide is an acceptable solution to seemingly insurmountable problems" (Portis et al., 2002, 811). Adolescence is a time when peer groups are paramount and parents are often pushed aside or no longer relied upon. The paradox, however, is that the adolescent needs the family more than ever to facilitate the development of the inner supports and provide the social supports for procuring the multitude of knowledge and skills that are necessary to transition successfully from adolescence to adulthood.

There are many circumstances in which adolescents consider suicide as an option. Adolescents who are most at risk of suicide are those who abuse drugs or alcohol, suffer from mood disorders, and experience interpersonal or conduct disorders. Research has shown that alcohol alone has been associated with more than one-half of adolescent suicides (Marcus, 1996). Other significant factors include personality disorders such as borderline or antisocial (Lester, 1993) and brain chemistry. Alterations in neurotransmitters are found in the postmortem brains of suicide victims. Puberty (age 12-14) also coincides with the first increase in the suicide rate as well as an increase in psychiatric illness and hormonal activity (Jamison, 1999).

51

Research shows that risk factors often occur in combinations. In other words, someone who is depressed and abusing drugs would be most at risk. Adverse life events along with risk factors also contribute to suicide risk. Breaking up with a girlfriend or boyfriend, divorce of parents, or physical and/or sexual abuse may contribute. Lester (1993) notes that suicidal adolescents more often than nonsuicidal adolescents experience some form of abuse, loss of parents during childhood and disturbed family relations. Often, parents of suicidal adolescents can be considered disturbed and may be suicidal themselves which further mandates that the entire family be involved in assessment and treatment. The parents' condition may increase the likelihood of depression in their children and, thereby, suicidal behavior.

Some people believe that more adolescents, especially boys, are successful at suicide, especially boys, because of the greater availability of guns along with "family disintegration, declining religious faith and greater economic challenges" (Marcus, 1996, 63). Girls, while attempting suicide more often, use less lethal methods such as drugs or cutting their wrists, and therefore, are less successful (Stone, 2001).

Many suicidal adolescents leave suicide notes. These notes are punctuated with anger, with more self blame than those of older persons, and with more evidence of disturbed interpersonal relationships (Lester,1993) Those adolescents who repeatedly attempt suicide are less educated, have had more school troubles and difficult parental situations as compared to first timers.

In summary, adolescents who contemplate suicide feel despair and misery. They cannot see any other life choices. They do not talk to their parents. They tend to isolate, do not talk about their feelings even with their friends. Death appears as the only way to alleviate their real pain. Yet, they often seek a way to escape and are not seeking death itself. Adolescents with suicidal behaviors are not well-connected to family and community.

Intervention

Health care professionals such as social workers, nurses and physicians learn to recognize that there are certain life problems that many adolescents face.

However, as noted above, adolescents are less likely to talk about their problems with professionals than any other age group (Granboulan et al, 2001, Pirkis et al, 2003). Compounding the difficulty is evidence that adolescents who attempt suicide have poor compliance records with outpatient treatment (Spirito et al., 2000). Lack of compliance makes it extremely difficult to assess whether a teen is suicidal.

Some believe that a number of suggested interventions can help prevent suicide in the adolescent. One intervention that is written about extensively is suicide prevention education (Eckert et al, 2003; King, 2001;Thatcher et al., 2001), which usually takes place in schools where both staff and students are taught to recognize when an adolescent may be suicidal. They learn to recognize signs of depression and drug abuse as well as to understand the risk factors that can lead to suicide. MacGowan (2003) refers to "gatekeeper training" that involves learning how to identify suicidal adolescents and how and where to obtain help. While some believe these programs are helpful, others doubt their ability to help those adolescents who are disconnected from schools and most at risk. Another preventive measure, though it has shown little effect in suicide rates, is the suicide or crisis hot line manned by trained volunteers. The idea behind the hot lines is that the caller remains anonymous. Thus, the adolescent feels in control of his/her destiny. One must note that the literature in this area is careful to point out that it is hard to measure whether any educational program does ultimately prevent suicides (Thatcher et al., 2002;Eckert et al., 2003).

Intervention by healthcare professionals is crucial to the prevention of suicide in adolescents. However, most often, it is a parent, teacher, or significant person in the adolescent's life who refers the adolescent to counseling or therapy. Because of the unique nature of adolescence and its appropriate life-stage tasks, adolescents are private, struggling with their desires to be independent, and distrustful of adults. This attitude obviously makes it more difficult for the social worker to develop a trusting relationship with the suicidal adolescent. Once a depressed or troubled adolescent agrees to talk with a social worker, it is important to ascertain the level of suicidal ideation through discussion and psychological testing. Psychological testing can give a somewhat objective measure of the adolescent's level of depression and sense of hopelessness (Donaldson et al., 2000). Utilizing discussion and testing together, the social worker can best assess the level of depression and suicidal thinking. At the same time, it is crucial to obtain a comprehensive family history and extend intervention to the entire family. Parent-family connectedness, emotional well-being, academic achievement, and perceived connectedness to school have all been identified as protective factors for attempting suicide irrespective of gender, racial, or ethnic groups (Borowsky et al, 2001). These findings strongly suggest the use of a family health approach in interventions with adolescents who are exhibiting suicidal behavior. If there is a history of depression and suicide in the family, there is a greater possibility that the adolescent will view suicide as a possible solution.

Once a social worker assesses that an adolescent is suicidal, s/he must decide how serious and/or imminent the threat is and how to intervene. Can this young man or woman be treated on an outpatient basis? Does s/he need medication? Or is the threat imminent enough that hospitalization is necessary? While attempting to answer these questions, the social worker also questions what his/ her duty is to the parents. Are the parents to be informed of concerns, even if the patient says no? Is the adolescent's autonomy to be respected above all else? Is the adolescent considered autonomous or impaired by his/her sense of hopelessness and depression? Thus, what on face value or prima facie seems to be a clear issue of good family intervention can become extremely complicated by the ethical responsibilities of the social worker.

Ethical Considerations

When social workers operate ethically, they act according to "moral principles adopted by an individual or group to provide rules for right conduct" (Corey, Corey & Calahan, 1993, p. 3). The National Association of Social Workers' (NASW) Code of Ethics provides broad guidelines for ethical social work practice (NASW, 1997). Values, which underlie ethical codes, refer to what one believes is good and desirable. Thus, social workers, to guide their thinking and actions, utilize both personal and professional ethics and values.

Ethical decisions made by helping professionals often involve issues that are complex and defy easy solutions. Almost all ethical decisions by nature involve choosing between two goods such as autonomy vs. duty to warn or autonomy vs. paternalism. When faced with a suicidal adolescent, the professional also faces a number of choices that force ethical decisions.

A rather substantial body of literature exists that discusses the ethical implications of working with suicidal adults. Yet, there is little literature about the unique ethical issues encountered in working with suicidal adolescents (MacGowan, 2003; Lester, 1999). So, it remains important here to discuss some of the ethical thinking around the issue of suicide and then to look at the specific decisions to be made when working with adolescents.

Well-known philosophers over the centuries have addressed the dilemma of intervening with suicidal individuals. Much of the thinking of these philosophers is reflective of their culture and their times. St. Thomas Aquinas, in the 1200s, argued that suicide was an offense against all, the self as well as society. Therefore, he argued for the absolute prohibition of suicide. David Hume, a Scottish philosopher of the 1700s, argued that suicide might serve the interests of one's self and others. Kant, well-known for his "categorical imperative"(to treat another as one would wish to be treated oneself—to act only if the act can be universal for all) and duty-based philosophy focused on the fundamental dignity that every rational person possesses (Rhodes, 1986). He argued that suicide is wrong because the principle of self-love always involves preserving life (Consculluela, 1995). More recently, Joel Feinberg (Beauchamp & Childress, 1996) views the respect for autonomy having precedence over protection of a person's welfare. Ringel, also writing more recently, supports suicidal preventive methods as a way to affirm human life believing that everyone "does not somewhere cherish the hope of being saved" (Beachamp & Childress, 1996, p.144). Szasz (1986, 1999) has written extensively on suicide, supporting the individual's liberty or right to suicide not because it is always a moral good but because the power of the state should not be used to prohibit or prevent people from taking their own lives. According to Szasz (1999), suicide is every person's ultimate right and therefore it is unethical for a professional to utilize coercion aimed at preventing the suicide. Yet, what if the person is not yet of adult age? As one can see, philosophers differ about the right and wrong of suicide. While none of the above specifically addresses suicide in children, all the above ethicists consider the following ethical principles in making their decisions.

Autonomy. Autonomy refers to a person's right to make his or her own decision about his or her life. Autonomy implies self rule or responsibility and derives from the Greek words "auto" meaning self and "nomos" meaning law or rule (Szasz, 1999). Social workers believe that the principle of autonomy is paramount in most situations. In fact, one of the primary values of social work, client self-determination, is derived from the principle of autonomy (Summers, 1989). However, it is a real challenge to determine with families when and how much autonomy to grant to adolescents. Even though laws and policies provide some guidelines and boundaries, many still consider this aspect of family life to be a slippery slope for both the families and the social workers.

Paternalism. Paternalism refers to the "intentional nonacquiescence or intervention in another person's preferences, desires, or actions with the goal of either avoiding harm to or benefiting the person" (Beauchamp, 1996, p. 127). While acting paternalistically is accepted in the health care field, the ethical commitment to autonomy requires that one reflect critically on the justification of any paternalistic intervention. Helping families and their adolescents determine the delicate balance between autonomy and paternalism that is beneficial to all family members is a formidable challenge. Not only do social workers have to be reflective, but families also have to learn to be thoughtful about how to use most effectively their parental rights with adolescents.

Principle of the Sanctity of Life. While this is more of a value than a principle, it becomes a critical factor in the decisions between autonomy and paternalism. Many hold the sanctity of life above all else. This would include issues of autonomy and confidentiality.

These principles then lead the social worker and families to crucial questions that must be answered when an adolescent is suicidal. Do the principles of respect for life and beneficence create an obligation for the social worker and family to prevent suicide? Does this obligation override any other obligation that would be based on the principle of respect for autonomy? When dealing with adolescents, might one say that an adolescent is autonomous when healthy, but not when s/he is depressed? Can s/he act in an autonomous fashion? Finally, if suicide is a protected moral right then the social worker would not have legitimate grounds for intervention unless an adolescent, by virtue of his/her age or depression, mental illness, or drug abuse is no longer viewed as autonomous.

To better understand these ethical issues a case will be presented here and discussed:

Sarah a 16-year-old adolescent female, has come to the mental health clinic because she feels depressed. Her mother is concerned about her and has encouraged her to talk with someone.

Sarah is a senior in high school and is applying to colleges. She is the eldest of seven children. Her father and mother both have Ph.D.s and her mother stays at home with the children. Her youngest sibling is almost two years old. Sarah has always been an excellent student, polite and well mannered, helping her mother with the other children. She also has a number of good girlfriends. She has never had a boyfriend and thinks of herself as ugly.

After meeting with Sarah twice it becomes clear that she is contemplating suicide. She has been cutting her wrists over the past month. She says it helps her to feel less anxious. She has thought about how and where she would kill herself. She has even thought about how the family will feel if she does. She is upset that her favorite teacher gave her a "bad" grade on a major paper. She never gets any "bad" grades. She feels that she has let her teacher down. She is also upset that her mother keeps having babies and then she has to help. Most upsetting to her, however, is that her parents are "making" her go to a religious college even though she has been accepted at the Ivy League school she really wants to attend. She believes that all the girls who attend this religious college do so to meet a man and get married. Since she feels that no young man would be interested in her, she knows that she will be miserable at this college.

The social worker who is working with Sarah has a number of ethical dilemmas to resolve. (One also has to keep in mind that some of these ethical dilemma present legal issues, which discussion is beyond the purview of this chapter.) The first dilemma involves the principle of confidentiality vs. the duty to warn. If Sarah has asked the social worker to maintain her confidentiality and not talk with her parents, then the social worker must decide whether to honor this request . The social worker must decide whether there is a greater duty to warn Sarah's parents of her suicidal intent and thus, breach confidentiality. If the social worker believes that Sarah is depressed, and therefore is no longer autonomous, or if the social worker believes that an adolescent should not be viewed as autonomous by virtue of age, then would it be ethically permissible to break the confidentiality and talk with her parents This argument relies on the belief that depression can be treated and relieved and that if this client gets better she will be glad to have been treated. It is acknowledged that breaking confidentiality may harm the social worker-patient relationship and Sarah may not trust the social worker and not return for needed help. Yet, the social worker's duty to provide no harm (malfeasance) may override Sarah's right to confidentiality.

The second ethical dilemma facing the social worker involves the issue of hospitalization. If the social worker believes that Sarah is imminently suicidal and should (according to good clinical practice) be hospitalized but Sarah does not want to be, the social worker is faced with an ethical dilemma that can be stated as paternalism vs. autonomy. Can the social worker override a patient's ethical right to autonomy if the patient is suicidal due to depression and hospitalize her against her will? Can she do so because Sarah is not yet 16? This is a very difficult dilemma that has been written about extensively when dealing with adults. It becomes more complicated when dealing with adolescents because of their young age. The question of at what age one has to be considered autonomous is difficult to answer. Perhaps, when children still live at home with their parents they should be viewed as nonautonomous. Some may argue from the belief that it is appropriate to violate a young person's immediate liberty if doing so will protect his or her autonomy later (Dworkin, 1989).

Thus, the two major ethical questions that the social worker must answer in this case are:

1.   Should the social worker inform/involve the family against an adolescent's wishes?

2.   When can a therapist commit a patient against his/her will?

A last question that is related but might be better dealt with at the beginning of a therapeutic relationship is the question of whether a social worker should insist on a "no- suicide contract?"

A no-suicide contract (NSC) is a therapeutic tool that encompasses the ethical issues discussed above. Can a social worker demand that Sarah sign a NSC? An NSC can be viewed as a way to avoid hospitalization while making it clear that if Sarah becomes suicidal, she agrees that the social worker can talk with her parents and commit her to a hospital if necessary. There is much discussion about NSC use with adults. Statistics do not show that an NSC is useful, and the question of coercion remains (Farrow and O'Brien, 2003; Reid, 1998). If the patient refuses to sign an NSC, then the relationship between social worker and patient is jeopardized. Finally, there is a large contradiction in asking depressed persons, who may not be autonomous, to sign an NSC as if they are autonomous and able to take control of their lives (Szasz, 1999).

Finally, answers to all these questions rest on how paternalistic a social worker is willing to be and how important it is to preserve the rights of a client (Howe, 1991). The ethical dilemmas intrinsic in this case present no "right" answer. It is the social worker's duty to choose the intervention that appears to be the most advisable ethically. In the case of Sarah, dealing with an adolescent who is depressed with a possible personality disorder, who does not have a long and recurrent history of depression, and who is young and cannot know whether she will get better, paternalistic interventions would be the most justified. A social worker, utilizing her or his best professional judgment, adhering to legal issues, and paying attention to both the family and ethical issues involved, would be acting in an ethical fashion toward his or her client if s/he breaks confidentiality to talk with parents about the patient's suicidal state and hospitalizes the client against the client's will if necessary.

Conclusion

Social workers must operate in an ethical manner and continue to search for the best practices in working with all kinds of vulnerable populations and problems. Suicidal adolescents and their families present social workers with many ethical dilemmas and practice challenges. All involve the issue of paternalism and the denial of client rights. Social workers must rely on their specific professional codes of ethics as well as their own personal values and ethics. This chapter suggests that social workers go beyond the traditional approaches to assessment and interventions with adolescents who exhibit suicidal behaviors by using a family health perspective. Although we as a society do not like to think or to talk about suicide, especially in regard to children and adolescents, we must address this problem in order to save young lives. This chapter represents a beginning discussion about a difficult mental health issue.

References

Allison, S., Roeger, L., Martin, G., & Keeves, J. (2001). Gender differences in the relationship between depression and suicidal ideation in young adolescents. *Australian and New Zealand Journal of Psychiatry, 35,* 498-503.

Ayyash-Abdo, H. (2002). Adolescent suicide: An ecological approach. *Psychology in the Schools, 39*(4), 459-475.

Beauchamp, T. & Childress, T. L. (1996) Moral problems and suicide intervention. In Beachamp, T. & Veatch, R. (Eds.). *Ethical issues in death and dying* (2nd ed.). pp. 127-130.

Borowsky, I. W., Ireland, M., & Resnick, M. D. (2001). Adolescent suicide attempts: Risks and protectors. *Pediatrics, 107*(3), 485-493.

Brent, D.A., Baugher, M., Bridge, J., Chen, T. & Chiappetta, L. (1999). Age-and sex-related risk factors for adolescent suicide. *Journal of the American Academy of Child Adolescent Psychiatry, 38*(12), 1497-1505.

Brernt, D.A. (1995). Risk factors for adolescent suicide and suicidal behavior: Mental and substance abuse disorders, family environmental factors, and life stress. *Suicide and Life-Threatening Behavior, 25*(Supplement), 52-63.

Brent, D. A., Perper, J. A. & Allman, C. J. (1987). Alcohol, firearms, and suicide among youth: Temporal trends in Allegheny County, Pennsylvania, 1960 to 1983. *Journal of the American Medical Association, 257,* 3369-3372.

Consculluela, V. (1995). *The ethics of suicide.* New York: Garland Publishing Inc.

Cory G/, Cory, M. & Callahan, G. (1993). *Issues and ethics in the helping professions.* Thousand Oaks, CA: Brooks/Cole Publishing Co.

Donaldson, D., Spirito, A. & Farnett, E. (2000). The role of perfectionism and depressive cognitions in understanding the hopelessness experienced by adolescent suicide attempters. *Child Psychiatry and Human Development 31*(2), 99-111.

Dworkin, Gerald (1997). *Mill's on liberty: Critical essays.* Lanham, Md.: Rowman and Littlefield Publishers.

Early, T. J. & GlenMaye, L. F. (2000). Valuing families: Social work practice with families from a strengths perspective. *Social Work, 45*(2), 118-131.

Eckert, T., Miller, D., DuPaul, G. & Riley-Tillman, T. (2003). Adolescent suicide prevention: School psychologists' acceptability of school-based program. *School Psychology Review, 32*(1), 57-76.

Egeland, J. A. & Sussex, J. N. (1985). Suicide and family loading for affective disorders. *The Journal of the American Medical Association, 254*(7), 915-918.

Erikson, E. (1968). *Identity: Youth and crisis.* New York: WW Norton & Co.

Farrow, T.L. & O'Brien, A.J. (2003) 'No suicide contracts' and informed consent: An analysis of ethical issues. *Nursing Ethics, 10*(2), 199-207.

Garofalo, R., Wolf, R. C., Wissow, L. S., Woods, E. R. & Goodman, E. (1999). Sexual orientation and risk of suicide attempts among a representative sample of youth. *Arch Pediatric Adolescent Medicine, 153,* 487-493.

Gould, M. S. & Kramer, R. A. (2001). Youth suicide prevention. *Suicide and Life Threatening Behavior, 31 (Supplement),* 6-31.

Granboulan, V., Roudot-Thoraval, F., Lemerle, S. & Alvin, P. (2001). Predictive factors of post-discharge follow-up care among adolescent suicide attempters. *Acta Psychiatrica Scandinavica, 104,* 31-36.

Howe, E. (1991). *Current perspectives in psychological, legal and ethical issues in children and families: Creation and conflict.* London: Jessica Kingsley Publishers, Ltd.

Jamison, K. R. (1999). *Night falls fast: Understanding suicide.* New York: Alfred A. Knopf.

Jennings, M. A. & Skibinski, G. (1999). Treating families through a family health perspective. In Pardeck, J. T. & Yuen, K. O. *Family health: A holistic approach to social work practice,* pp. 45-59. Westport, CT: Auburn House. .

King, K. A. (2001). Developing a comprehensive school suicide prevention program. *Journal of School Health, 71*(4), 132-137.

Lester, D. (1993). *The cruelest death: The enigma of adolescent suicide.* Philadelphia: The Charles Press.

MacGowan, M.J. (2003). Prevention and intervention in youth suicide. In Allen-Meares and Fisher (Eds). *Intervention with children and adolescents: An interdisciplinary perspective* (pp.282-310). Boston, MA: Allyn and Bacon

Marcus, Eric (1996). *Why suicide?* San Francisco: Harper.

Mohler, B. & Earls, F. (2001) Trends in adolescent suicide: Misclassification bias? *American Journal of Public Health, 91*(1), 150-153.

National Association of Social Workers. (1997). Code of Ethics of the National Association of Social Workers. Washington, DC: Author.

NIMH (2003). In harm's way: Suicide in America. Retrieved July 25, 2004, from http://www.nimh.nih.gov/publicat/harmaway.cfm.

Pardeck J.T. & Yuen, F.K.O. (1999). Family health: A holistic approach to social work practice. Westport, CT: Auburn House.

Pelkonen, M. & Marttunen, M. (2003). Child and adolescent suicide: Epidemiology, risk factors, and approaches to prevention. *Pediatric Drugs 5*(4), 243-265.

Pirkis, J. E., Irwin, C. E., Brindis, C. D., Sawyer, M. G., Friestad, C., Biehl, M., et al. (2003). Receipt of psychological or emotional counseling by suicidal adolescents. *Pediatrics, 111*(4), 388-393.

Portes, P. R., Sandhu, D. S. & Longwell-Grice, R. (2002). Understanding adolescent suicide: A psychosocial interpretation of developmental and contextual factors. *Adolescence, 37*(148), 805-814.

Reid, W. H. (1998). Promises, promises: Don't rely on patients' no suicide/no-violence "contracts." *Journal of Practical Psychiatry and Behavioral Health, 4*(5), 316-318.

Rhodes, Margaret L. (1986). *Ethical dilemmas in social work practice.* Boston: Routledge & Kegan Paul.

Rowan, A. B. (2001). Adolescent substance abuse and suicide. *Depression and Anxiety, 14*, 186-191.

Spirito, A., Boergers, J. & Donaldson, D. (2000). Adolescent suicide attempters: Post-attempt course and implications for treatment. *Clinical Psychology and Psychotherapy, 7*, 161-173.

Stone, G. (2001). Suicide and attempted suicide. New York, NY: Carol & Graf Publishers, Inc.

Summers, A. B. (1989). The meaning of informed consent in social work. *Social Thought, 15*(3), 128-140.

Szasz, T. S. (1986). The case against suicide prevention. *American Psychologist, 41*, 806-812.

Szasz, T. S. (1999). Rethinking suicide. *The Freeman, 49*, 41-42.

Thatcher, W. G., Reininger, B. M., & Drane, J. W. (2002). Using path analysis to examine adolescent suicide attempts, life satisfaction, and health risk behavior. *Journal of School Health, 72*(2), 71-77.

Chapter 5
Adolescent Substance Abuse and the Family Health Social Work Perspective
Stephen J. Brannen

Introduction

Over the past decade there has been a growing concern within the medical, legal, and human services communities regarding the increased usage of substances by adolescents (Johnston, O'Malley, & Bachman, 1995) and the decreased age of first usage by adolescents (Reich, Cloninger, Van Eerdevegh, Rice, & Mullaney, 1988). Data provided in the Monitoring the Future Survey (Johnston, O'Malley, & Bachman, 1995), an annual survey of high school seniors, show that during the first half of the 1990s there was an increase in adolescent substance abuse. Over the past several years, this use has leveled off (Substance Abuse and Mental Health Services Administration, 2001), albeit at higher prevalence rate established by the increased usage pattern of the early- to mid-1990s.

Patterns of Abuse

The Substance Abuse and Mental Health Services Administration (SAMHSA, 2001) reports that approximately 8.9% of youths aged 12 to 17 had used inhalants. In this same age category, the rate of current illicit drug use for boys (9.8%) and girls (9.5%) was consistent (2001). Boys had a slightly higher rate of marijuana use than girls (7.7% compared to 6.6%), while girls were more likely to use psychotherapeutic drugs non-medically than boys (3.3% compared to 2.7%).

Approximately 27.5% (9.7 million) of American adolescents reported drinking alcohol within the month prior to being surveyed. SAMHSA (2001) estimates that of this figure, 6.6 million (18.7%) considered themselves binge drinkers and another 2.1 million (6%) identified themselves as heavy drinkers. The rates reported in 2000 household surveysremained consistent in the latter half of the 1990s. Consistent with previous reports, males aged 12 to 20 were more likely than the females to engage in binge drinking (21.3% compared to 15.9%) (SAMHSA, 2001).

While the number of new adolescent marijuana users and cigarette smokers decreased in the late 1990s, the number of adolescents using psychotherapeutics non-medically increased from 1999 to 2000. Youths aged 12 to 17 have reported an increase in usage from 78,000 in 1985 to 722,000 in 1999. Consistent with past Household Surveys, adolescents age 12 and over indicated that it was quite easy to obtain illicit substances including marijuana, cocaine, crack, heroin, and LSD (SAMHSA, 2001). Unfortunately, the rates of use of most drugs in 2000 remain higher among youth and young adults than among mature adults. Over all in 2000, about half (49%) of the illicit drug users were under the age of 26; 83% of hallucinogen users, 62% of inhaling users, 32% of heroin users, 3% of cocaine users, and 45% of non-medical psychotherapeutic users were under the age of 26.

Gender

The rate of current illicit drug use among adolescents is very similar for boys and girls (9.8% compared to 9.5% respectively). While boys are slightly more likely to use marijuana than girls (7.7% compared to 6.6%), girls are more likely to use psychotherapeutics non-medically than boys (3.3% compared to 2.7%). At the end of the 1990s there were no significant changes in the rate of current illicit drug use for other males or females aged 12 to 17 (SAMHSA, 2001).

Age of First Use

Youths age 12 to 17 constituted approximately two thirds of the new users of marijuana, with young adults aged 18 to 25 constituting almost the remaining third. These rates are the highest ever reported for both the adolescents and young adults (SAMHSA, 2001). Youths age 12 to 17 represent the largest group of new cocaine users. While in 1991 there were approximately 92,000 new cocaine users, in 1998 the number of new cocaine initiates among youth had risen to 339,000 (SAMHSA, 2001).

In 1999 there were a reported 1.4 million new users of hallucinogens (i.e., LSD and PCP). Of this figure, 669,000 were found in the age category 12 to 17 years and an additional 604,000 were between 18 and 25 (SAMHSA, 2001).

In 1999 there were approximately 1.5 million new users of psychotherapeutics (including stimulants, tranquilizers, and sedatives), a figure that has been increasing since the mid-1980s. Unfortunately, youths aged 12 to 17 constituted the majority of the increase, from 78,000 in 1985 to 772,000 in 1999.

In 1998, 5.1 million people initiated the use of alcohol in this country, the highest number of new users recorded since data have been maintained. The largest single group represented in this rise is youths age 12 to 17 with 3.4 million new drinkers, approximately 67% of all new drinkers. This 3.4 million new adolescent users represents about 15% of the total youth population in United States (SAMHSA, 2001).

Race/Ethnicity

The 2000 National Household Survey on Drug Abuse shows that the rates of current illicit drug use for the major racial/ethnic groups were 6.4% for whites, 5.3% for Hispanics, and 6.4% for African-Americans. The rates were highest among the American Indian/Alaska natives (14.8 percent) and the lowest among Asians (2.7%). The increased use of the illicit drugs by African-Americans demonstrates a shift in usage patterns from previous surveys, which found that in 1991 African-American youths reported lower rates of psychoactive drug use than any other racial or ethnic group (SAMHSA, 2001).

67

College Age Youths

Peterson, Nisenholz, & Robinson (2003) describe the cohort of college-age adolescents as "probably one of the best documented groups of adolescent alcohol abusers" (p. 73). They argue that college students drink an estimated four billion cans of beer each year. Eigan (1991) found that, on a yearly basis, college students spend more money on alcohol consumption than on textbooks. Wechsler, Kuo, Lee, & Dowdall (2000a), in a major survey of college drinking, found that of under-aged students, 63% had drunk in the 30 days prior to being surveyed. When compared with college students of legal age, they drank on one fewer occasion, but had more drinks per occasions than students. In a second study, Wechsler and his associates found that over 44% of college students surveyed were binge drinkers, while 19% were abstainers. These researchers observed that the number of frequent binge drinkers increased significantly from 1994 to 1999 (Wechsler, Lee, Kuo, & Lee, (2000b).

While alcohol remains the substance of choice for college-age adolescents, the rate of illicit drug use remains slightly (above 18%). These rates are consistent for those who are full-time college students as well as for part-time students, students in other grades, or non-students (SAMHSA, 2001).

Pattern of Abuse by Geographic Location

According to the National Household Survey on Drug Abuse, the rates of illicit drug abuse were very similar across the counties. While rates of 8% were found in less urbanized non-metropolitan counties, the rate for use in large metropolitan areas was 9.4%. In the urbanized metropolitan counties the use rate was 11.5% (SAMHSA, 2001).

Consequences of Adolescent Substance Abuse

While identifying the extent of the drug-abuse problem facing our youth today is important, a far more important issue facing this country is the role that drugs play in psychiatric disorders, motor vehicle accidents, suicides, homicides, violence, drowning, delinquency, and unprotected sexual behavior (Crumley, 1990; Dembo, Williams, Schmeidler, Wish, Getreu, & Berry, 1991; DiClemente, 1990; Kaminer, 1994; Kaminer & Bukstein, 1998), as well as the impact it has all on the individual, family, and society (Children's Defense Fund, 1991; National Institute of Justice, 1994).

Mortality

The Centers for Disease Control (CDC) reports that unintentional injuries, including motor vehicle accidents, are the leading cause of death in adolescents, accounting for 29% of all deaths. It is estimated that 50% of these deaths are related to the consumption of alcohol by adolescents (CDC, 1998).

Sexually Risky Behaviors

Adolescents who abuse alcohol and drugs are more likely than others to engage in sexual relationships and other risky sexual behaviors. MacKinzie (1993), in a survey of Massachusetts adolescents, found two thirds reported having had sexual intercourse, 64% reported having had sex after using alcohol, and 15% reported having sex after using drugs. McKenzie also found that substance use decreases an individual's selection of sexual partners, increases the number of sexual partners, and increases the likelihood of the adolescents' practicing risky sexual behaviors, thereby increasing the likelihood of developing a sexually transmitted disease (STD).

An additional consequence of substance use for females is unwanted pregnancy. According to the National Institute of Drug Abuse (NIDA), an estimated 4.9% of females under the age of 18 annually give birth to a live infant. Of these young women, 12.4% used alcohol and 21.9% smoked cigarettes during their pregnancies. An additional 5.7% used illicit drugs (marijuana or cocaine) while they were pregnant, thus increasing the risks of fetal alcohol syndrome, miscarriage, and restricted fetal growth during the pregnancy. All these conditions result in substantial economic and health-care costs to society each year (Winters, 1999).

Delinquency and Crime

The relationship between conduct disorder and substance use among adolescents has been consistent over time (Crowley & Riggs, 1995). Dembo (1996) found that many youths entering the juvenile justice system have an array of problems ranging from emotional, psychological, and educational difficulties to physical abuse, sexual victimization, and substance- use disorders (SUD). Currently, most adolescents presenting to residential treatment facilities have been mandated to treatment by the criminal justice system (Jainchill, 1997).

Studies have confirmed that conduct disorder and aggressive behavior are typically associated with SUDs (Huizinga & Elliot, 1981; Milin, Halikas, Meller, & Morse, 1991). Use of substances such as alcohol, amphetamines, and PCP is believed to increase the likelihood of increased aggressive behavior in adolescents (Moss & Tarter, 1993).

Developmental Problems

Substance use has been linked with adolescents' lack of success in accomplishing normal developmental tasks such as dating, marrying, bearing and raising children, establishing a career, and building interpersonal relationships (Baumrind & Moselle, 1985; Havighurst, 1972; Newcomb & Bentler, 1989). Conversely, adolescents' use of alcohol and drugs is believed to hinder their emotional and intellectual growth and impair identity development (Havighurst, 1972).

Substance Abuse and the Family-Health Social Work Perspective

As Daly (2003) suggested, the traditional method of assessing and treating adolescent substance (alcohol) abuse does not appear capable of addressing all facets of the problem. Daley's argument that "the role of the family in the treatment process has ranged from being peripheral to being a major causal destructive force to needing concurrent or separate treatment" (p. 113) may well be true for those entering drug abuse interventions as well. While many clinical programs give lip service to the inclusion of families in the treatment process, typically these programs continue to be singularly focused on the individual, treating the family as an adjunct or afterthought. Rather than basing assessment and intervention strategies upon a standardized nosological system designed for adults and adapted for adolescents that focus the vast majority of attention on interpersonal factors, the family health perspective offers a holistic approach to the assessment of adolescent substance abusers.

Family health social work practice focuses its assessment and intervention strategies not solely on the individual, but includes the micro and macro levels (Pardeck, 2003). While interpersonal characteristics are addressed using a strengths perspective (Saleebey, 1997), the family health social work perspective stresses the need to identify problems and weaknesses not only within the individual, but also within the community and society as a whole (Yuen, 2003).

Pardeck and Yuen (1999) describe family health as "manifested by the development of, and continuous interaction among, the physical, mental, emotional, social, economic, cultural and spiritual dimensions of the family which results in the holistic well-being of the family and its members" (p. 1). As Daly (2003) has argued, the existing models of substance-abusing family interventions recognize that family functioning is distorted and has a negative impact on family members when the family is substance-abuse centered. The family health model further postulates that each of the seven dimensions is negatively impacted as the substance abuse and its sequelae weaken both the individual and the family.

Assessment Using the Family Health Perspective

In assessing for adolescent substance abuse/dependence using the family health perspective, the physical, mental, emotional, social, economic, cultural, and spiritual dimensions must be thoroughly evaluated. While historically social workers have relied upon the clinical interview, the use of this subjective process, however critical, has its limitations and must be supplemented with objective procedures. In fact,Winters (1999) argues for the use of two methods in assessing adolescent substance use disorders: self-report questionnaires, and structured or unstructured interviews. Winters argues that these methods can yield "an accurate, realistic understanding of the teenager and the problems he is experiencing"(p. 22). Not only does a well-designed assessment process help in identifying the presence of a substance-use problem, but also, implemented correctly, it can provide important insights into the adolescent's motivation and readiness to engage in and benefit from intervention (Winters, 1999). Each of the seven dimensions will be discussed with recommendations provided on how appropriately to assess it.

Assessment of the Physical Dimension (History of Substance Use)

The assessment interview is the most significant and central feature in the screening/assessment process. The interview allows the social worker to address and target specific questions to the seven dimensions of the family health perspective. Margolis (1995) recommends that two specific series of interviews be conducted: one with the adolescent alone and one jointly with a parent. Certainly, the adolescent's history of substance use, including over-the-counter and prescription drugs, alcohol, cigarettes, and illicit drugs must be the central focus of the assessment process. It is important to note the age of first use; frequency, length, and pattern of use; method of ingestion; treatment history; and signs and symptoms of substance- use disorders, including loss of control and preoccupation with the use of substances. In addition, parents can provide information concerning a family history of substance use and psychiatric illnesses, as well as provide a comprehensive medical and developmental history. However, specific information concerning substance use should be addressed with the adolescent during that interview. Finally, Margolis recommends that a mental status examination be conducted with special attention paid to sudden unexplained mood swings as well as unexplained difficulties with the judgment and insight. Winters (1990) suggests that additional interviews may be necessary to develop a clear understanding of the history of the adolescent substance use pattern. It might be beneficial to collect data using structured or semi-structured interviews with family members and others important to the user (Winters, 1990).

In addition, screening and rapid assessment instruments (RAIs) can provide objective verification of information collected in the clinical interview. Several instruments have demonstrated excellent psychometric properties and are useful in assessing multiple dimensions identified using the family-health perspective.

For initial screening of adolescents abusing alcohol, the Michigan Alcohol Screening Test (MAST) (Selzer, 1971) has been long recognized as the gold standard. This 24-item scale is easy to administer, score, scale, and interpret. When used as a screening tool, scores of three and less are indicative that the

72

client does not consider themselves to have a problem with alcohol; a score of four suggests that the client may be a problem drinker, while scores over five and above are indicative that the person does have an alcohol dependency. Craig (2004) suggests that when using the MAST during treatment planning, it is useful to segment problematic responses into categories. Questions 1-5 pertain to psychological and attitudinal issues; questions 2,4,7,9, and 16-18 pertain to alcoholic symptoms; questions 2,3,6, and 10-12 relate to interpersonal relations affected by drinking; questions 8 and 19-22 pertain to treatment for alcoholism; questions 13-15 pertain to vocational problems; while questions 23 and 24 regard legal problems.

The Drug Abuse Screening Test (DAST) (Skinner, 1982), much like the MAST, is a self-report measure that is a brief and easy to administer, score, scale, and interpret. Consisting of 20 items, the DAST provides information on the consequences of drug use and abuse and can be used as part of an interview or as a self-report measure. Like the MAST, the DAST can be used in a variety of clinical settings. Unlike the MAST, the DAST does not have established cutoff scores. However, Skinner recommends that a score of six or higher is indicative of a drug problem. Additionally as the scores increase the implication is that individual's drug problem is more severe.

The Personal Experience Inventory (PEI) (Winters & Henley, 1989), a self-administered instrument, was designed to be used with adolescents. It develops information concerning patterns of substance use well as behaviors frequently associated with substance use. It consists of 276 questions contained in two parts, the Chemical Involvement Problems Severity section and the Psychosocial section. Requiring a reading level of sixth-grade, it typically requires 45-60 minutes to complete.

The Problem Oriented Screening Instrument for Teenagers (POSIT) was developed as a screening instrument by the National Institute on Drug Abuse (NIDA) in an effort to identify potential problem areas in need of further in-depth assessment. The instrument, consisting of 139-item "yes/no" questions, assesses substance use and abuse, physical health, mental health, family relations, peer (social) relations, educational status, vocational status, social skills, leisure/recreation, and aggressive behavior/delinquency. The POSIT takes approximately 20-30 minutes to complete and two to five minutes to hand score (Rahnert, 1991).

The Drug Use Screening Inventory (DUSI) (Tarter, 1990) is a 159-item, self-administered instrument that documents adolescent involvement with a variety of drugs and quantifies the severity of consequences associated with drug use. The instrument flags problem areas in the following areas: substance use behavior, behavior patterns, health status, psychiatric disorders, social skills, family system, schoolwork, peer relationships, leisure, and recreation. The DUSI requires approximately 15-20 minutes to complete.

The Teen Addiction Severity Index (T-ASI) provides a relatively brief assessment instrument developed for use when an adolescent is being admitted into care for substance-use-related problems. It consists of an objective face-to-face interview that yields usage and severity ratings. Life areas assessed using the system include chemical use, school status, employment/support, family relationships, peer/social relationships, legal status (involvement with criminal justice program), and psychiatric status (Kaminer, Buckstein, & Tarter, 1991; Kaminer, Wagner, Plummer, & Seifer, 1993).

Finally, given the high prevalence of risk-taking behaviors while under the influence of substances (Leigh & Stall, 1993), it is critical that social workers working with adolescents receive training on HIV/AIDS prevention, education, and referral. The assessment must contain specific questions regarding high-risk sexual behavior, such as needle sharing, while the agency must have established policies and procedures on referral of adolescents to agencies that can provide further in-depth assessment for HIV/AIDS, while still maintaining client confidentiality. Obviously, questions regarding high risk behaviors should be addressed only during the individual interview with the adolescent.

Assessment of the Family

Many experts consider substance abuse to be a family problem (Craig, 2004). In fact, Liddle and Dakof (1995) consider the family to be the key element in all aspects of screening, assessing, and treating adolescents for substance abuse disorders. Ott and Totter (1998) state that family organization and interaction patterns contribute to both the etiology and maintenance of substance abuse. There is strong evidence that the transmission of alcohol across generations is strongly influenced by family member attitudes and rituals regarding the use of substances and the meanings attached to use (Steinglass, Bennett, Wolin, & Reiss, 1987). To address family historical information, the joint clinical interview with the adolescent and a parent or knowledgeable family member can be of tremendous importance. Furthermore, instruments such as the POSIT, DUSI, and T-ASI mentioned above contain specific items addressing the family system and family relationships.

The characteristics of families of substance abusers have been extensively studied. These   include the fact that alcohol and drug abuse occur more often in addict families; substance-abusing families are engaged more frequently in conflict; alliances between and among family members are explicitly understood; caregivers of the substance abuser tend to show a great degree of attachment and symbiosis with the abuser; substance-abusing families experience premature, untimely, unexpected, and tragic deaths than non-abusing families; and substance-abusing families experience more trauma including divorce, separation, accidents, deaths, and sexual trauma than other families (Alexander & Dibb, 1975, 1977; Harbin & Maziar, 1975). These characteristics are believed to not only maintain the addictive behavior, but also to maintain the stability of the family or one of the family relationships (Craig, 2004).   How substance use precipitates family dysfunction and how family problems may trigger substance use are two areas that need to be addressed (Ott & Tarter, 1997). While there are several family-assessment instruments available to clinical social workers, two that have demonstrated effectiveness in identifying family coping and resiliency and family functioning are widely used in both research and clinical practice.

In addressing resiliency and family coping, the Family-Crisis Oriented Personal Evaluation Scales (F-COPES) has been developed (McCubbin, Larson, & Olson, 1982). This 30-item, self-report instrument based on the McCubbin's

Resiliency Model assesses the manner in which a family internally handles difficulties and problems between its members and the manner in which the family externally handles problems or demands emerging outside its family boundaries but which nonetheless affecting the family unit and its members.

The Family Assessment Device (FAD-III) (Epstein, Baldwin, & Bishop, 1983), a 60-item self-report measure, assesses family functioning along six domains: problem solving, communications, family member roles, affective responsiveness, affective involvement, and behavioral control. In addition, the FAD-III provides an overall measure of functioning called the general functioning scale. The FAD-III is extremely useful with substance-abusive families as a tool in identifying issues that contribute to the family's dysfunction.

Finally, social workers involved in the assessment and treatment of adolescent substance abusers should reconsider the traditional definitions of family, for they no longer are applicable for many within our society. According to the family-health perspective (Pardeck, 2003), a family is "a system of two or more interacting persons who are either related by ties of marriage, birth, or adoption, or well-chosen to commit themselves to each other in unity for the common purpose of promoting the physical, mental, emotional, social, economic, cultural, and spiritual growth and development of the unit and each of its members" (p. 9).

To assist in the development of the family identity and structure, the Genogram (Guerin & Pendagast, 1976) and Ecomap (Hartman, 1978) are extremely useful and widely adopted tools within social work practice. While a genogram identifies family structure in the micro level, the ecomap is useful in assessing stressors and functioning which occur at the micro, macro, and mezzo levels.

Assessment of the Mental Dimension

A mental health history should be an integral part of the adolescent-substance-abuse assessment. This history should focus on any indications of depression, suicide attempts, attention-deficit disorders, anxiety disorders, and behavioral disorders, as well as any previous history of mental health or psychiatric interventions (Winters, 1999). Kaminer and Buckstein (1998) suggest that one fourth to one half of adolescents abusing substances can be dually diagnosed with a depressive disorder; 50 to 80% can be diagnosed with conduct disorder; and up to 40% may present with co-morbid anxiety disorders. In addition to the development of a well-rounded history, a thorough mental status examination (MSE) should be conducted (Margolis, 1995). In the MSE, the clinician should pay attention to sudden, unexplained mood swings as well as unexplained difficulties with the judgment. The MSE must contain questions regarding "intent to harm self or others."

However, in many cases, the adolescent may require evaluation beyond the scope of a clinical social worker's practice. In these cases, it is important for the social worker to be familiar with the various psychological tests, testing protocols, and methods of referring to a testing psychologist for evaluation.

Assessment of the Emotional Dimension

As has been mentioned above, adolescents involved in substance abuse will very frequently present with co-morbid emotional disturbances. These disturbances may include mood disorders (anxiety and depression), conduct disorders, difficulties in peer relationships, difficulties in family relationships, attention-deficit disorder, etc. Because mood disorders are the most commonly occurring disorder, it is important that the social worker become familiar with evaluating the adolescent for the presence of these disorders. In the primary care arena a commonly used assessment device to screen for depression is the Zung Self-Depression Screening Scale (SDS). The SDS is a 20-item instrument developed to examine three basic aspects of depression: pervasive affect, physiological concomitants, and psychological concomitants. The SDS consists of 10 items worded symptomatically positive and 10 items symptomatically negative. Items on the SDS were specifically selected to tap one of the three aspects of depression described above and include cognitive, affective, psychomotor, somatic, and social-interpersonal items. The SDS takes only a matter of minutes to be administered, scaled, and scored. The SDS is readily available for use by clinical social workers.

77

Derogotis (1983) developed the Symptom Checklist 90 (SCL-90) to be used as a screening device for emotional and psychological disturbances and adolescents and adults. The SCL-90 is highly useful in assessing for the presence of anxiety disorders as well as other mood disorders. In addition to the SCL-90, there are shorter derivatives. The most commonly used of these is the Brief Symptom Inventory (BSI) (Derogotis, 1983). In addition, Hudson (1992) developed the WALMYR Assessment Scales. Among the numerous scales in the WALMYR Assessment Scales packet is one that specifically assesses for anxiety disorders, as well as a scale that measures peer relationships.

Assessment of the Social Dimension

Peer relationships are a significant impactor on the initiation, development and maintenance of substance abuse in adolescents (Kaminer & Buckstein, 1998). In fact, peer influences play the crucial role in the process of involvement for all substances of abuse: tobacco, alcohol, and illicit drugs. Research has shown that most substance use occurs due to social influences and can be attributed to the adolescent's subculture and peer group (Jessor & Jessor, 1977; Kaminer & Buckstein, 1998). Jessor and Jessor (1977) found that the most consistent finding in substance abuse research is the relationship between an adolescent's substance abuse behavior and the concurrent use by his or her peers.

Given this, it is important that the clinical interview and the joint parental interview contain specific items requesting information regarding school history (including academic and behavioral performance, and attendance problems); peer relationships, interpersonal skills, and gang involvement and neighborhood environment; juvenile Justice involvement in delinquency, including the types and incidence of behavior and attitudes towards that behavior; leisure time activities, including recreational activities, hobbies, and interest. The POSIT, DUSI and T-ASI all contain items that specifically address several of these items.

Assessment of the Cultural Dimension

Aoki, Delgado, de Miranda, Hatchett, Magiste, Mattingly-Langlois, and Whitford (1994) argue that the days when the traditional substance abuse client is middle-class, middle-aged, Caucasian, and male are over. They suggest that treatment programs and professionals need to understand, acknowledge, and appreciate the diversity in their clientele in order to respond to the individualized needs of their clients. The social worker practicing in the substance-abuse arena needs to develop not only an appreciation for diversity, but also an assessment and intervention strategy that addresses the uniqueness of the individual within their cultural context. Ashenberg-Straussner (2001) describes this as ethnocultural competency, the ability of a clinician to function effectively in the context of ethnocultural differences. Tirado (1998) found that ethnocultural competency not only influenced client-clinician communications and trust, but was additionally a crucial component in the effective provision of substance abuse services and the retention of clients.

Noting the difficulty that adolescents generally experience in relationship to adult figures, using an ethnocultural perspective would be beneficial in working with adolescents of culturally diverse groups. Furthermore, an important aspect of ethnocultural assessment is understanding the client's family, its structure, role expectations within the family, and the relationship of substance abuse to these characteristics (Ashenberg-Straussner, 2001). Within the social work arena, strengths-based practices focusing on assessing what an individual wants, coupled with the skills, resources, and resiliencies found within the individual and the community have proven effective in working with clients from disparate cultures (van Wormer & Davis, 2003).

The Culturally Informed Functional Assessment (CIFA) Interview (Tanaka-Matsumi, Seiden, & Lam, 1996) provides a conceptual framework and practical guideline for culturally informed assessment and treatment planning. The CIFA Interview was designed to facilitate case formulation with clients who is cultural backgrounds were different than that of the clinician. The interview includes eight steps, each successively focusing on a specific assessment issue from the perspective of the client, the clients family and/or significant others, and the culture or sub-culture. The goals are to define the clients problems correctly, demonstrate respect for the client culture, and negotiate the change activities. It is designed to accommodate culturally excepted norms for role behavior, the cultural-role definition of behaviors, expectations regarding interventions, and culturally sanctioned change agents.

Assessment of the Spiritual Dimension

Spirituality, an aspect frequently discussed in the treatment literature (van Wormer, 2003) is rarely attended to using traditional screening and assessment protocols. While spirituality is considered to be a cornerstone of many self-help groups (AA, NA, etc.), Royce (1989) found that a vast majority of clients receiving substance abuse treatment complained that their spiritual needs were not addressed within the traditional treatment programs. Carrol (1999) suggests that the 12 Steps of Alcoholics Anonymous offer a guide toward increasing self-knowledge, sharing with others, and reached a higher level of consciousness. Finally, O'Connell (1999) found that for those in addiction recovery, approaches offering enhancement of spiritual awareness increased the sense of purpose in the addict's life. O'Connell argues that the client's attitude toward a sense of spiritual well-being should be routinely evaluated and addressed during the intervention in recovery process. And finally, as van Wormer and Davis (2003) state, "There is a growing recognition among providers of culturally specific programs ... that spiritual believes offer a great resource. Clients from other ethnic groups, as well, can benefit from tapping into this often-overlooked resource . . ." (p. 107).

Assessment interviews should include items which addresses the extent that spiritualism plays in the role of the client. However, as Yuen (2003) points out, care must be given to ensure that the concept of spiritualism is differentiated from both faith and religion. Consequently, the definition adopted by the family health perspective, spirituality is defined as

> a drive, need, power or capacity . . . . It is that non-material, mysterious aspect of the person; the ground of one's being that strives for meaning, union with universe, and all things .... It seeks to transcend the self, to discover meaning and purpose in the world. It is expressed in form-in the connectedness with nature, in personality, and culture-in the experience of the aesthetic, and in religion or in any form that seeks related us to the infinite. (p. 2)

Faith is considered to be "an intersystem . . . which relates to one's transcendent or ultimate reality, for the theistic believer, God" (Joseph, 1997, p. 2). Religion is "the organized, outward expression of that connectedness and meaning" (Raines, 1997, p. 8). It is quite possible that someone can be very spiritual but have no affiliation with any religious organization, and equally possible that a very religious individual could not be spiritual (Yuen, 2003).

As Yuen (2003) states, spirituality and/or spiritual growth is a very difficult construct not only to define, but also to measure in a clinical setting. Yuen offers several alternatives to measurement of this difficult construct: utilizing a single subject designed to measure the frequency, intensity, and duration of behavioral indicators of spiritual gains identified as important to the client; and qualitative methods such as use of a reflective report or journal which will be discussed with the clinical social worker. However, there are few empirically validated instruments that have proven utility in this arena. One such instrument that may be beneficial in the assessment of the adolescents is the Spiritual Well-being Scale (Paloutizan & Ellison, 1982). While the 20-item scale addresses both spirituality and religiosity, it has demonstrated a utility if clinicians utilize individually endorsed items during the assessment process. Obviously a great deal of effort needs to be placed into empirically validating this component of assessment and treatment.

Assessment of the Economic Dimension

There are two factors that should be addressed during the clinical interview regarding the family-health perspective's economic dimension as it applies to adolescent substance users: reduced achievement motivation and the disparity between substance costs and availability of resources to the adolescent substance user.

Jessor (1987) found that adolescent substance abusers are less likely to attend church, are less likely to value academic performance and/or perform well academically, and are more likely to have reduced believes in the generalized expectations, norms, and values of society. As a consequence of their substance use, they are less likely to actively seek out employment.

Clinical social workers must address the issue of the incongruity between the cost of continuing substance use any ability of the adolescent to pay for the drugs to be used. The question must be addressed regarding where the adolescent obtains the funds with which to purchase drugs. Certainly, there is evidence to support that as substance use increases, delinquent behavior increases. In fact, Kaminer and Bukstein (1998) argue that these activities may be routed in the identity-creating process of increased substance use/dependence.

Motivation for Change

Over the past several years there has been a shift from the conservative (medical) model of treatment that emphasized type of treatment setting, length of stay, and the 12-Step dominated approach to and approach that emphasizes matching the stage of treatment to the individual needs of the client (Kaminer & Bukstein, 1998). The critical element in the stage-matched treatment protocols is the determination of a client's motivation to change. Measuring client motivation is not a singular task and requires that each of several dimensions of motivation the evaluated. These include the client's perception of self-efficacy, the import that the client places on the eliminating substance use, the clients readiness to change, evaluating the decisional balance, and determining the motivations for continued use of substances (Miller, 1999). The benefits of employing motivational enhancement techniques include inspiring motivation to change, preparing clients to enter treatment, engaging and retaining clients in treatment, increasing client participation in involvement with treatment, improving treatment outcomes, and encouraging a rapid return to treatment if substance-abusive tendencies and symptomology return (Miller, 1999). To this end, several instruments have been developed that assist in the measurement of a client's motivation to change. These include the Brief Situational Confidence Questionnaire (BSCQ) (Sobell, 1996), the Readiness to Change Questionnaire (Treatment Version) (RTQ-TV) (Heather, Rollnick, & Bell, 1993), the Situational Confidence Questionnaire (SCQ-39) (Annis & Graham, 1988), the Stages of Change Readiness and Treatment Eagerness Scale (SOCRATES), (Miller & Tonigan, 1996), the Alcohol (and Illegal Drugs) Decisional Balance

Scale and the University of Rhode Island Change Assessment Scale (URICA) (McConnaughy, DiClemente, Prochaska, & Velicer, 1983).

Intervention Strategies

As the substance abuse field has become more sophisticated, it has consistently integrated conflicting theories and approaches to treatment, as well as incorporating research findings into the treatment process. As a result, many changes have emerged with a new view of motivation, with associated strategies to enhance client motivation moving to the forefront. Whereas in the past treatment has focused on deficits and psychopathology within the individual, today there is a greater emphasis on identifying, enhancing, and using clients' strengths and competencies. In the past, clients received standardized treatment, regardless of their problems or the severity of their substance dependence. Today treatment is client centered, based upon individual client needs, and the result of a careful and thorough assessment process. While in the past a diagnosis or disease defined the client and potentially became a dehumanizing attribute of the individual, in the substance abuse arena today there is a trend to avoid labeling individuals. Clinicians use a motivational style to avoid branding clients with names, especially those who may not agree with a diagnosis or do not see a particular behavior as problematic (Miller, 1999).

This shift in thinking about motivation and substance abuse intervention includes the concept that change is a process rather than an outcome. As a natural outgrowth, the change process has been conceptualized as a sequence of stages through which people typically progress as they think about, initiate, and maintain new behaviors (Prochaska & DiClemente, 1984). Their Trans-Theoretical Model (TTM) envisions a process that involves five specific stages of change: precontemplation, contemplation, preparation, action, and maintenance.

Summary: from Assessment to Treatment Using the Family Health Perspective

This chapter presented an overview of the extent of adolescent substance abuse in the United States. Specific substances of abuse and their prevalence rates were discussed in an effort to establish the need for the implementation of a multi-variable, holistic assessment based upon the family health social work perspective. Specific screening and assessment methodology were provided and discussed that addressed the seven dimensions of the family health social work perspective. In addition, the assessment of and adolescent's motivation to change was discussed, as well as a stage-of-change model for treatment of adolescent substance abuse. While the Trans-Theoretical (Stages of Change) Model has been widely adopted in the treatment of a wide variety of addictive and problematic behaviors in adults, to date there have been no studies supporting its use with adolescent substance abusers. Future research should focus on the development of treatment/intervention strategies with adolescents and using this model, coupled with a thorough assessment utilizing the family health social work perspective.

References

Aoki, B., Delgado, M., de Miranda, J., Hatchett, R., Magiste, E., Mattingly-Langlois, K., & Whitford, L. (1994). Cultural sensitivity: Treatment for diversity. In K.C. Winters & Zenilman, J.M. (Panel Co-Chairs). *Simple screening instruments for outreach for alcohol and other drug abuse and infectious diseases* (pp. 58-63). Substance Abuse and Mental Health Services Administration (SAMHSA). Rockville, MD: U. S. Department of Health and Human Services.

Alexander, B.K., & Dibb, G.S. (1975). Opiate addicts and their parents. *Family Process, 14,* 499-514.

Alexander, B.K., & Dibb, G.S. (1977). Interpersonal perception in addict families. *Family Process, 16,* 505-525.

Annis, H.M., & Graham, J.M. (1988). *Situational confidence questionnaire.* Toronto, ON: Addiction Research Foundation.

Ashenberg-Straussner, S.L. (2001). *Ethnocultural factors in substance abuse treatment.* New York: The Guilford Press.

Baumrind, D., & Moselle, K.A. (1985). A developmental perspective on adolescent drug abuse. *Advances in Alcohol and Substance Abuse, 4,* 41-67.

84

Centers for Disease Control and Prevention. (1998). *Leading causes of mortality and morbidity and contributing behaviors in the United States, 1998.* Retrieved March 22, 2002 from http://www.cde.gov/nccdphp/dash/ahsumm/ussumm.htm .

Children's Defense Fund. (1991). *The adolescent and young adult fact book.* Washington, DC: Children's Defense Fund.

Carrol, M.M. (1999). Spirituality and alcoholism: Self-actualization and faith stage. *Journal of Ministry in Addiction & Recovery, 6*(1), 67-84.

Connors,G.J., Maisto, S.A., & Zywiak, W.H. (1998). Understanding relapse in the broader context of posttreatment functioning. *Addiction, 91*(Supplement), 173-189.

Craig, R.J. (2004). *Counseling the alcoholic and drug dependent client.* Boston, MA: Allyn & Bacon.

Crowley, T.J., & Riggs, P.D. (1995). Adolescent substance use disorder with conduct disorder and co-morbid conditions. In E. Rahdert, and Czechowicx, D. (Eds.). *Adolescent drug abuse: Clinical assessment and therapeutic interventions* (pp. 49-111). National Institute on Drug Abuse (NIDA) Research Monograph Series, No. 156. Rockville, MD: National Institute on Drug Abuse,.

Crumley, F.E. (1990). Substance abuse and adolescent suicidal behavior. *Journal of the American Medical Association, 263,* 3051-3056.

Daly, J.G. (2003). Navigating family health in families with alcohol abuse. In F.K.O. Yuen, Skibinski, G.J., & Pardeck, J.T., *Family health social work practice: A knowledge and skills casebook* (pp. 113-145). New York: The Hayworth Social Work Practice Press.

Dembo, R. (1996). Problems among youths entering the juvenile justice system, their service needs, and innovative approaches to address them. *Substance Abuse and Misuse, 31*(1), 81-94.

Dembo, R., Williams, L., Schmeidler, J., Wish, E.D., Getreu, A., & Berry, E. A prospective study of high risk youth. *Journal of Addictive Diseases, 11*, 5-31.

Derogotis, L.R. (1983). *SCL-90: Administration, scoring and procedures manual II* (rev.). Towson, MD: Clinical Psychometric Research.

DiClemente, C.C. (1990). The emergence of adolescents as a risk group for human immunodeficiency virus infection. *Journal of Adolescent Research, 5,* 7-17.

DiClemente, C.C., & Prochaska, J.O. (1998). Toward a comprehensive trans-theoretical model of change: Stages of change in addictive behaviors. In W.R. Miller, & Heather, N. (eds.). *Treating addictive behaviors* (2nd ed.). New York: Plenum Press.

Eigan, L. (1991). *Alcohol practices, policies, and potentials of American colleges and universities.* Substance Abuse and Mental Health Services Administration (SAMHSA). Rockville, MD: U. S. Department of Health and Human Services.

Epstein, N.B., Baldwin, L., & Bishop, D. (1983). The McMaster Family Assessment Device. *Journal of Marital and Family Therapy, 9,* 213-228.

Guerin, P.J., Jr., & Pendagast, E.G. (1976). Evaluation of family systems and genograms. In P.J Guerin Jr. (Ed.) *Family therapy: Theory and practice.* New York: Gardner Press.

Harbin, H.T., & Maziar, H.M. (1975). The families of drug abusers: A literature review. *Family Process, 14,* 411-431.

Hartman, A. (1978). Diagrammatic assessment of family relationships. *Social Casework, 59,* 465-476.

Havighurst, R.J. (1972). Nurturing the cognitive skills in health. *Journal of School Health, 42*(2), 73-76.

Heather, N., Rollnick, S., & Bell, A. (1993). Predictive validity of the Readiness to Change Questionnaire. *Addiction, 88,* 1667-1677.

Hudson, W.W. (1992). *The WALMYR Assessment Scales scoring manual.* Tempe, AZ: WALMYR.

Huizinga, D., & Elliot, D.S. (1981). *A longitudinal study of drug use and delinquency in a national sample of youth: An assessment of causal order*

(Project Report No. 16, A National Youth Study). Boulder, CO: Behavioral Research Institute.

Jainchill, N. (1997). Therapeutic communities for adolescents: The same and not the same. (161-177). In G. De Leon (Ed.). *Community as method: Therapeutic communities for special populations and special settings.* (pp. 161-177). Westport, CT: Praeger.

Johnston, L.D., O'Malley, P.M., & Bachman, J.G. (1995). Prevalence of drug use among 8th, 10th, and 12th grade students. *National survey results all in drug use from the Monitoring the Future Study, 1975-1994. Volume I, secondary school students.* Rockville, MD: National Institute on Drug Abuse.

Jessor, R (1987). Problem-behavior theory, psychosocial development and adolescent problem drinking. *British Journal of Addiction, 82*, 331-342.

Jessor, R., & Jessor, S.L. (1977). *Problem behavior and psychosocial development: A longitudinal study of youth.* New York: Academic Press.

Joseph, M.V. (1997). Toward the future: call, covenant, mission. *Society for Spirituality and Social Worker Newsletter, 4*(1), 8-9.

Kaminer, Y. (1994). *Adolescent substance abuse: a comprehensive guide to theory and practice.* New York: Plenum.

Kaminer, Y., & Bukstein, O.G. (1998). Adolescent substance abuse. In R.J. Frances and Miller, S.I. *Clinical textbook of addictive disorders* (2nd ed.) (pp. 346-373). New York: The Guilford Press.

Kaminer, Y., Bukstein, O.G., & Tarter, R.E. (1991). The teen-addiction severity index: Rationale and reliability. *International Journal of Addictions, 26*, 219-226.

Kaminer, Y., Wagner, E., Plummer, B., & Seifer, R. (1993). Validation of the teen addiction severity index (T-ASI). *American Journal of Addiction, 2*, 250-254.

Leigh, B.C., & Stall, R. (1993). Substance use and risky behavior for exposure to HIV. Issues in methodology, interpretation, and prevention. *American Psychologist, 48*(10), 1035-1045.

Liddle, H.A., & Dakof, G.A. (1995). Family-based treatment for adolescent drug use: State of the science (pp. 218-254). In E. Rahdert, and Czechowiz, D. (Eds.). *Adolescent drug abuse: Clinical assessment and therapeutic interventions.* Rockville, MD: National Institute on Drug Abuse.

MacKenzie, R.G. (1993). Influence of drug use on adolescent sexual activity. *Adolescent Medicine: State of the Art Reviews, 4*(2), 112-115.

Margolis, R. (1995). Adolescent chemical dependence: Assessment, treatment, and management. In A.M. Washton, (Ed.). *Psychotherapy and substance abuse: A practitioner's handbook* (pp. 394-412). New York: The Guilford Press.

McConnaughy, E.A., DiClemente, C.C., Prochaska, J.O., & Velicer, W.F. (1983). Stages of change in psychotherapy: Measurement and sample profiles. *Psychotherapy: Theory, Research and Practice, 20,* 368-375.

McCubbin, H., Larson, A., & Olsen, D.H. (1982). (F-COPES) Family coping strategies. In: Olsen, D.H., McCubbin, H.I., Barnes, H., Larson, A., Muxen, M. & Wilson, M. (Eds). *Family Inventories: Inventories used in a national survey of families across the family life cycle* (pp. 101-119). St. Paul, MN: Family Social Science, University of Minnesota.

Milin, R., Halikas, J.A., Meller, J.E., & Morse, C. (1991). Psychopathology among substance abusing juvenile offenders. *Journal of the American Academy of Child and Adolescent Psychiatry, 30,* 569-574.

Miller, W.R. (1999). *Enhancing motivation for change in substance abuse treatment.* Substance Abuse and Mental Health Services Administration (SAMHSA). Rockville, MD: U. S. Department of Health and Human Services.

Miller, W.R., & Tonigan, J.S. (1996). Assessing drinkers' motivation for change: The Stages of Change Readiness and Treatment Eagerness Scale (SOCRATES). *Psychology of Addictive Behaviors, 10*(2), 81-89.

Moss, H.B., & Tarter, R.E. (1993). Substance abuse, aggression, and violence: What are the connections? *American Journal of Addiction, 2,* 149-160.

National Institute of Justice. (1994). *Drug use forecasting: 1993 annual report on juvenile arrestees/detainees. Research in brief.* Washington, DC: National Institute of Justice.

Newcomb, M.D., & Bentler, P.M. (1989). Substance use and abuse among children and teenagers. *American Psychologist, 44*(2), 42-48.

O'Connell, D.F. (1999). Spirituality's importance in recovery cannot be denied. *Alcoholism & Drug Abuse Weekly, 11*(47), 5.

Ott, P.J., & Tarter, R.E. (1998). Comprehensive substance abuse evaluation. In R.J. Frances and Miller, S.I. *Clinical textbook of addictive disorders* (2nd ed.) (pp. 35-70). New York: The Guilford Press.

Paloutizan, R.D., & Ellison, C.W. (1982). Loneliness, spiritual well-being in the quality-of-life. In L.A. Peplau & Perlman, D. (Eds.). *Loneliness: a sourcebook of current theory, research & therapy (pp. 224-237).* New York: Wiley Interscience Publication.

Pardeck, J.T. (2003). An overview of family health social work practice. In F.K.O. Yuen, Skibinski, G.J., & Pardeck, J.T. *Family health social work practice: A knowledge and skills casebook* (pp. 3-16). New York: The Hayworth Social Work Practice Press.

Pardeck, J.T., & Yuen, F.K.O. (Eds.) (1999). *Family health: A holistic approach to social work practice* (p. 1). Westport, CT: Auburn House.

Peterson, J.V., Nisenholz, B., & Robinson, G. (2003). *A nation under the influence: America's addiction to alcohol.* Boston: Allyn & Bacon.

Prochaska, J.O., & DiClemente, C.C. (1984). *The trans-theoretical approach: Crossing traditional boundaries of therapy.* Homewood, IL: Dow Jones-Irwin.

Prochaska, J.O., & DiClemente, C.C. (1992). Stages of change in the modification of problem behaviors. In M. Herson, Eisler, R.M., & Miller,R.W (Eds.). *Progress and behavior modification (Vol. 28)* (pp. 183-218). Sycamore, IL: Sycamore Publishing Co.

89

Rahdert, E.R. (Ed.). (1991). *The adolescent assessment and referral system manual* (DHHS Publication No. ADM 91-1735). Rockville, MD: National Institute on Drug Abuse.

Raines, J. (1997). Spiritual assessment: An initial framework. *Society for Spirituality and Social Worker Newsletter, 4*(1), 8-9.

Reich, T., Cloninger, P., Van Eerdevegh, J.P., Rice, J.R., & Mullaney, J. (1988). Secular trends in the familial transmission of alcoholism. *Alcoholism: Clinical and Experimental Research, 12,* 458-464.

Royce, J.E. (1989). *Alcohol problems and alcoholism: A comprehensive survey* (Rev. ed.). New York: Free Press.

Saleebey, D. (1997). *The strengths perspective in social work practice* (2nd ed). White Plains, NY: Longman.

Selzer, M. (1971). The Michigan Alcohol Screening Test: The quest for a new diagnostic instrument. *American Journal of Psychiatry, 127,* 1653-1658.

Skinner, H.A. (1982). The Drug Abuse Screening Test. *Addictive Behaviors, 7,* 363-371.

Sobell, L.C. (1996). Bridging the gap between science and practitioners: The challenge before us. *Behavior Therapy, 27,* 297-320.

Steinglass, P., Bennett, L., Wolin, S., & Reiss, D. (1987). *The alcoholic family.* New York: Basic Books.

Substance Abuse and Mental Health Services Administration (2001). *Summary of findings from the 2000 national household survey on drug abuse.* Rockville, MD: Substance Abuse and Mental Health Services Administration (SAMHSA). Rockville, MD: U. S. Department of Health and Human Services.

Tanaka-Matsumi, J., Seiden, D.Y., & Lam, K.N. (1996). The culturally informed functional assessment (CIFA) interview: A strategy for cross-cultural behavioral practice. *Cognitive and Behavioral Practice, 3,* 215-233.

Tarter. R.E. (1990). Evaluation and treatment of adolescent substance abuse: A decision tree method. *American Journal of Drug and Alcohol Abuse, 16,* 1-46.

Tirado, M.D. (1998). *Monitoring the managed care of culturally and linguistically diverse populations.* Vienna, VA: National Clearinghouse for Primary Care Information.

van Wormer, K., & Davis, D. R. (2003). *Addiction treatment: A strengths perspective.* Pacific Grove, CA: Brooks/Cole.

Wechsler, H., Kuo, M., Lee, H., & Dowdall, G. (2000a). Environmental correlates of under age alcohol use and related problems of college students. *American Journal of Preventive Medicine, 19*(1), 24-29.

Wechsler, H., Lee, J., Kuo, M., & Lee, H. (2000b). College binge drinking in the 1990s: A continuing problem. Results of the Harvard School of Public Health 1999 college out all study. *Journal of American College Health, 48*, 199-210.

Winters, K.C. (1990). The need for improved assessment of adolescent substance involvement. *Journal of Drug Issues, 20*(3), 487-502.

Winters, K.C. (1999). *Treatment of adolescents with substance use disorders. Substance Abuse and Mental Health Services Administration (SAMHSA).* Rockville, MD: U. S. Department of Health and Human Services.

Winters, K.C. & Henley, G. (1989). *Personal Experience Inventory Test and Manual.* Los Angeles: Western Psychological Services.

Yuen, F.K.O. (2003). Family health practice with the spiritually diverse person. In F.K.O. Yuen, Skibinski, G.J., & Pardeck, J.T. *Family health social work practice: A knowledge and skills casebook* (131-144). New York: The Hayworth Social Work Practice Press.

Zung, W. K. (1965). A self-rating depression scale. *Archives of General Psychiatry, 12*, 63-70.

Chapter 6

The Most Despised--Juvenile Sexual Offenders: How They and Their Families Can Be Healthy

Hal Agler

Juvenile sexual offenders (JSO's) are one of the most despised classes of clients treated for their misbehaviors. Even those trained to work with varied issues in therapy may have problems based on biases they internalize. Marked preferences are seen for clients who have been abused themselves because they are perceived as having an apparent reason for their acting out versus those that have no abuse history.

The latter group is also more likely to be seen simply as criminals beyond the reach of therapy (Carone & LaFleur, 2000). To demonstrate the size of the problem, the number of treatment facilities specializing in offending behaviors increased from 20 in 1982 to 650 in a little over a decade (Lakey, 1995). Shockingly, treatment programs for offenders below age 12 now numbers over 300 (Ryan, 1999).

Despite the difficulties arising during treatment of JSO youth, involvement and reunification with the family are still primary goals. However, the nature of the crimes committed make accomplishment of these goals more difficult than for other delinquent youth. Adding to this problem is the fact that roughly 39% of the victims of juvenile sexual offenders are siblings or other children living in the same home (Veneziano, 2000). Also, the problematic nature of the families that are often the homes for youthful offenders require specialized, intensive interventions.

The treatments for these adolescents are very important since half of the adult offenders began in their teens with a median age of 14 years (Lakey, 1995; Salter, et al, 2003). The pattern of offending is also carried into adulthood as the use of coercion or age of the victims is often determined during the teenage years (Caputo, Frick, & Brodsky). Further, more than half of all reported male child victims and 30% of female child victims were abused by a teen (Ryan, 1999). In a study of the general population, 3-4% of youths from 15-20 years old have committed a sexual offense. This translates into 500,000 yearly offenses, which is in sharp contrast to 16,000 arrests during the same period (Bischof, Stith, & Whitney, 1995). Another important fact is that 62% of victims of youthful offenders are under 12 years old and 44% are under six years old (Veneziano, 2000).

Juvenile offenders are heterogeneous group with diverse needs and a wide range of intellects and abilities. However, many share attributes that will be important to consider when working with them individually and when evaluating a return to their families as safe, contributing members. Many of the youths exhibit inadequate intimate relationships and expect rejection. This is caused most often by attachment problems in infancy, which are triggered by neglect or mistreatment by significant caregivers (Barbaree, Marshall, & Hudson, 1993; Salter, et al, 2003). Ryan (1999) states this lack of childhood attachment to a caregiver causes the breakdown in the formation of empathic interrelations and the lack of understanding of others' feelings by abusers. The development of angry, coercive, and aggressive behaviors may also serve to gain the attention of unresponsive caregivers and will be carried over into all their relationships (McCormack, Hudson, & Ward, 2002). There is also a strong correlation of interfamilial violence as a common precursor of sexual misconduct with up to 79% of offenders reporting involvement in different forms of physical and emotional abuse (Caputo, Frick, & Brodsky, 1999).

Other shared traits that can contribute to the etiology of sexually abusive behaviors are feelings of inadequacy, low self esteem, atypical erotic fantasies, poor social skills, personal sexual abuse history, poor school performance, inadequate impulse control, substance abuse, and expansive instability in their personal environments (Lakey, 1994). There are few positive mediators with correspondingly low numbers of positive influences identified in the lives of offenders (McCormack, Hudson, & Ward, 2002). Offenders share a propensity to deny the offenses and to show a lack of remorse for the damage that may be caused and a distinct lack of victim empathy, even if they were previously victimized themselves. The offender is also highly likely to be completely self absorbed, focused only on fulfilling personal wants and needs. There is also a high correlation with other non-sexual offenses because of the effects of impulsiveness and boredom (Lakey, 1994).

Estimates of the amount of JSO's that have experienced sexual abuse vary by the sample, but estimates range from 40% to a high of 90%. When all types of abuse are factored in, very few abusive youth would not be represented (Ryan, 1999). The offender, in a study in 2000 by Veneziano, demonstrated a strong predilection to repeat the abuse suffered at a younger age. Those studied were very likely to repeat the same offenses to a peer of a similar age of onset for their own abuse. This leads to the conclusion that the JSO is often reenacting the abuse experienced in childhood.

Adolescent offenders typically view their families as unsupportive of them or their independence, as placing little emphasis on intellectual and cultural pursuits, and as not being active together or sharing recreational experiences. Similarly, the family is more likely to be bound by strict rules with little communication or open expression (Bischof, Stith, & Whitney, 1995). Since the abuser has experienced a high level of problems, it will be necessary to intervene at several levels for effective treatment. Family health is paramount because of the myriad concerns in this realm. Individual treatment cannot be successful by itself without addressing the issues within the family such as intergenerational abuse and victimization, substance problems, and neglect (Gray, Busconi, Houchens, & Pithers, 1997).

Treatment for an offender on an outpatient basis can last over 18 months, and more severe cases of abuse may require long-term residential treatment (Kahn, 1997). Whichever course of treatment is chosen, the involvement of the family will be necessary to insure the highest level of functioning for all the members. Therapeutic goals for the sexually abusive youth include definition of abuse in their daily lives, recognition of associated patterns of abuse, development of skills to interrupt these patterns, acknowledgement of the risk for continued offending, development and demonstration of empathy, and the ability to develop and maintain safe, appropriate relationships (Ryan, 1999). These skills are not developed in a vacuum and should be part of individual and family therapy. The family is still a family even if immediate reunification is blocked for any reason. Overall functioning, individuation, improved relationships, and the healing of other family members can all be facilitated through family therapy (Rich, 2000). However, the high likelihood of adolescent diagnoses (such as 73% with Conduct Disorder, 41% with ADHD, and 27% with Oppositional and Defiant Disorder) make it clear these clients will be problematic in treatment and will test even a seasoned therapist (Gray, Busconi, Houchens, & Pithers, 1997).

The first reaction of the family is often to minimize the behaviors of the child in question, believing "boys will be boys" or that it was simply youthful experimentation instead of a sexual offense (Marshall, Laws, & Barbaree, 1990). It is important to jar the family out of the complacency of denunciation and accept the seriousness of the offenses. The parents must support the truth and not accept the offender's early minimizations and denial (Kahn, 1997; Swenson, Henggeler, Schoenwald, 1998). An early attempt to shield the perpetrator or family from outside scrutiny or ridicule can become a difficult hurdle to overcome as treatment progresses.

The route to treatment can be an early indicator of what is to come. If the family brought the offense to the attention of appropriate authorities, they take it seriously and are in a position to support the victim. If the offender is turned in through outside reporting, the family's reaction will need to be assessed fully before treatment begins (DiGiorgio-Miller, 1998).

Rich (2000) provides some general guidelines to use in family therapy with youthful offenders and the rest of the family:

- Both custodial parents should attend sessions including a stepparent or live-in acting as a parent figure.
- If parents are divorced, the most involved parent who will be providing support should attend.
- If the divorced parents are both involved, family therapy should be offered to both sets of parents.
- If offered to two sets of parents, blended sessions should be attempted if possible.
- Any siblings should have the cognitive ability to deal with the sexual behaviors to be discussed.
- These siblings should be present for the disclosure phase if this will lead to support for the victim or perpetrator.
- Victims should not engage in family therapy until sessions are working toward victim clarification.
- Extended family members such as grandparents should also be present if they play a role in parenting or raising the children.
- Therapy should begin with those members that are willing and available and then involve other family members as they become more willing.

The dynamics of the offender's family will also play an important role in determining the direction of therapy. The overall denial of the behavior, even with the admission of the perpetrator, is a common hurdle. Minimization of the serious impacts of the behavior can also be a significant problem. The family may also be looking for someone else to blame to relieve the offender of responsibility. The victim will often be the repository for this behavior, even if the victim is a sibling. Friends, school, television, and special situations or circumstances can all be utilized to minimize personal responsibility. Parents and siblings may also have had suspicions or knowledge of abuse and have chose to ignore it for some reason, hoping the problem would take care of itself. This is often accompanied with parental guilt and shame. Family secrets about intergenerational abuse, incest, or inappropriate exposure to sex at a young age, such as viewing pornography, may also be shared by the family members (Imber-Black, 1993). Family environmental factors such as secrets, myths, and sexual taboos dramatically increase failure rates in treatment and recidivism after discharge (Baxter, Tabacoff, Tornusciolo, & Eisenstadt, 2003). Feelings of stigmatization can follow, further blocking progress. Parents can feel helpless about why and how the abuse occurred and use this to cover more intense feelings about the offense. If the victim is in the home, another common problem occurs when family members take sides between the two parties and do not understand the role of victim and perpetrator. Also, the victim's emotional needs may be overlooked because of the focus on the offender's legal and therapeutic problems. The parents, forced into this situation, are likely to give mixed messages to family members as they work at sorting out the truth.

Important milestones in family therapy begin with a thorough assessment of the family and introduction to the goals and regimens employed in JSO treatment (Lundrigan, 2001). The family is also oriented to the process of family therapy as an intervention in the course of treatment. Pertinent information is disseminated to the family at this time that corresponds with the work the youth will be doing in sessions. The important elements of the treatment process and treatment plan are discussed, and support is provided to help the family through the roadblocks they will face.

The next step is for the youthful offender to clarify what was done in a disclosure meeting with his or her parents. The full discussion of the events will be a very difficult task for the youth who is used to hiding feelings and avoiding contact and isolating from the family (Kahn, 1997). This meeting is best completed as the individual has become involved in treatment and has a clear understanding of the behaviors exhibited that were problematic. The meeting will aid the parents in seeing the true extent of the perpetrator's offenses (Lundrigan, 2001). Victim clarification is another important part of this meeting as the relationships among the offender, victim, and family members are delineated. Young siblings should not be involved in this meeting so they are not unnecessarily traumatized or sexualized by the information. However, it is suggested that older siblings could benefit from participation to understand the need for safety and to help hold the offender accountable in the family setting (Rich, 2000).

As formal treatment begins to make sufficient headway, the prevention of relapse becomes a major focus of individual and family interventions (Lundrigan, 2001). Formulation of the relapse safety and prevention plan is the last step before reunification and is one of the most important parts of the treatment process. The plan involves all members of the family by definition and is the document that holds the offender to the steps necessary to maintain in-home safety for the family and out-of-the-home safety for community members. At this point, the offender and family members clarify rules and responsibilities to minimize the risk for relapse. It is vitally important for the youth to be able to identify the behaviors that caused the offense and discontinue them, such as grooming potential victims. This type of maintenance behavior helps get the perpetrator close to a vulnerable individual. It is also vitally important for the therapist to recognize possible future victims that can be in the home or neighborhood during this phase (Gray, Busconi, Houchens, & Pithers, 1997).

If the youth has offended children who are much younger, a portion of the plan will deal with eliminating contact with potential victims through restrictions on play, babysitting, and going to places where victims could be found such as playgrounds. Further risks such as riding the bus, being unsupervised at school, staying overnight at another's home, and going on dates and outings may be included. The installation of monitoring devices such as door alarms and neighbor notification may also be necessary components. Other high-risk behaviors such as deviant stimulation through the use of pornography or substance use would also be addressed. Virtually any part of the adolescent's life can and should be addressed in the plan (Kahn, 1997). Even with a strong, comprehensive plan, the reality is that the offender should never be trusted to be in a dangerous situation again.

This is the place where formal risk assessment takes place. It is here that referral sources such as child welfare agencies and juvenile justice jurisdictions ask if the child is safe to return to the home environment or needs a more restrictive environment based on continued signs of future abusive behavior such as deviant fantasies or thinking errors or distortions that will allow the offender to excuse future sexual misconduct. The involvement of all those involved in the treatment process is used to help answer this single question. Factors such as understanding empathy, personal responsibility for actions, motivation for ongoing self control, and the quality of current relationships are common items to be examined during the process.

After the child is formally discharged from treatment, the final meetings with the family should provide encouragement as well as cautions against complacency (Lundrigan, 2001). If the child is able to go directly home, the safety plan and everyone's responsibilities to maintain it should be reviewed. Future commitments for ongoing treatment will also be necessary to support behavioral changes and to help assess any future risks. Studies of recidivism among youthful sexual offenders vary from 3% in a one-year follow-up to nearly 20% in a five-year longitudinal study. Further, 40% of the youth participated in at least one non-sexual offense after treatment discharge (Witt, Bosely, & Hiscox, 2002). Again, a combination of factors goes into determining any future behavior problems and the ability to return to a life with the family.

References

Barbaree, H., Marshall, W., & Hudson, S. (1993). *The juvenile sexual offender.*
New York: The Guilford Press.

Baxter, A., Tabacoff, R., Tornusciolo, G., & Eisenstadt, M. (2003). Family
secrecy: A comparative study of juvenile sex offenders and youth with
conduct disorders. *Family Process, 42*(1), 105-116.

Bischof, G., Stith, S., & Whitney, M. (1995). Family environments of adolescent sex offenders and other juvenile delinquents. *Adolescence, 30*(117), 157-170.

Caputo, A., Frick, P., & Brodsky, S. (1999). Family violence and sexual offending: The potential mediating role of psychopathic traits and negative attitudes towards women. *Criminal Justice and Behavior, 26*(3), 338-356.

Carone, S. & LaFleur, K. (2000). The effects of adolescent sex offender abuse history on counselor attitudes. *Journal of Addictions & Offender Counseling, 20*(2), 56-64.

DiGiorgio-Miller, J. (1998). Sibling incest: Treatment of the family and offender. *Child Welfare, 77*(3), 335-346.

Gray, A., Busconi, A. Houchens, P., & Pithers, W. (1997). Children with sexual behavior problems and their caregivers: Demographics, functioning, and clinical pattern. *Sexual Abuse: A Journal of Research and Treatment, 9* (4), 267-290.

Imber-Black, E. (Ed.) (1993). *Secrets in families and family therapy.* New York: W. W. Norton & Co.

Kahn, T. (1997). *Pathways guide for parents of youth beginning treatment.* Brandon, VT: The Safer Society Press.

Lakey, J. (1994). The profile and treatment of male adolescent sex offenders. *Adolescence, 29*(116), 755-761.

Lundrigan, P. (2001).*Treating youth who sexually abuse: An integrated multi-component approach.* New York, NY: The Haworth Press.

Marshall, W., Laws, D., & Barbaree, H. (Eds.) (1990). *Handbook of sexual assault: Issues, theories, and treatment of the offender.* New York: Plenum Press.

McCormack, J., Hudson, S., & Ward, T. (2002). Sexual offender's perceptions of their early interpersonal relationships: An attachment perspective. *The Journal of Sex Research, 39*(2), 85-93.

Rich, P. (2000). *Juvenile sexual offenders: Understanding, assessing, and rehabilitating.* Hoboken, NJ: John Wiley& Sons, Inc.

Ryan, G. (1999). Treatment of sexually abusive youth. *Journal of Interpersonal*

Violence, 14(2), 422-436.

Salter, D., McMillan, D., Richards, M., Talbot, T., Hodges, J., Bentovin, A., Hastings, R., Stevenson, J., & Skuse, D. (2003). Development of sexually abusive behavior in sexually victimized males: A longitudinal study. *Lancet, 361*(9356), 471-476.

Swenson, C., Henggeler, S., & Schoenwald, S. (1998). Changing the social ecologies of adolescent sexual offenders: Implications of the success of multisystemic therapy in treating serious antisocial behavior in adolescents. *Child Maltreatment, 3*(4), 330-338.

Veneziano, C. (2000). The relationship between adolescent sex offender behaviors and victim characteristics with prior victimization. *Journal of Interpersonal Violence, 15*(4), 363-374.

Witt, P., Bosely, J., & Hiscox, S. (2002). Evaluation of juvenile sexual offenders. *The Journal of Psychiatry and Law, 30,* Winter, 569-592.

Chapter 7

Strategies in Family Health Practice: Inclusion of Play Therapy
Glenda Short

Family Health focuses on a holistic state including the physical, mental, emotional, social, economic, cultural and spiritual dimensions of the family (Pardeck and Yeun, 1999). Within this model, health is defined as "a state of holistic well-being which constitutes meaningful connections within the natural and human world" (Pardeck, Yeun, Daley, and Hawkins, 1998 p.29). Since play enhances and involves all areas of well-being, play, or the ability to play, is connected to all aspects of the Family Health Model. Research shows us that all aspects of play (biological, recreational, psychological, cognitive, social, cultural, spiritual, and physical health) translate into economic savings by investing self in play activities (Freud, 1920; Erikson, 1950, 1963; Axline, 1947; Mead, 1934; Piaget, 1951; Landreth, 1982; Landreth, 1993; Schaefer, 1993; Bratten and Landreth, 1995; Glass, 1986; Leblanc and Ritchie, 2001; Elliot and Pumfrey, 1972). The use of play therapy to achieve the functions of a family health model needs further exploration and understanding. Individuals within the family affect the health issues of each family member, particularly the physical and emotional functioning (Akamatsu, Stephens, Hobfoll, and Crowther, 1992). And all family members are positively or negatively affected by another member's health status.

The definition of family is an important one when discussing the Family Health Model, particularly when you begin to form conclusions about how members are affected when another member suffers poor health or enjoys good health in any of the holistic areas of this model. Pardeck and Yuen (2001) define family as a system of two or more persons who are related in some way or who are committed to a relationship. This commitment focuses on the common purposes of promoting each family member's physical, mental, emotional, social, economic, cultural, and spiritual growth and development. A variety of research confirms that this definition fits our society (Cheal, 1993, Wisensale, 1992; Zimmerman, 1992). Further, other types of families are now identified and differ from the traditional family make-up that has dominated our thinking. Blended or reconstituted families, binuclear families, communal families, gay/lesbian families, and cohabitating families are mentioned in the literature. Most researchers agree about the primary focus of families, regardless of what complexities are found. The family is the principle system by which knowledge, values, attitudes, roles, and habits are transmitted (Thornton, Chatters, Taylor, and Allen, 1990; Kochanska, 1990; Peterson and Rollins, 1987). Each of these factors is a vital component that helps to define an individual's physical and mental health status.

As in any system, there are transactional patterns that establish the functioning of family tasks. These functions are identified as the activities that are needed to move toward common purposes in all areas of family health. Pardeck and colleagues (1998) identified six functions that families establish and act on for the benefit of each member. These functions also help to stabilize the overall health of family members and society: 1) physical care and economic security, 2) the mental growth and development of the family members, 3) emotional nurturance, 4) socialization, 5) cultural transformation, and 6) spiritual growth. These functions have not been clearly developed within the Family Health Model in terms of examples and ways that families accomplish them.

The Power of Play across Developmental Stages

A variety of strategies and techniques can be employed to complete any or all of these functions and move toward a healthier family. Play, however, is one of the most potent strategies. According to William C. Menninger (1967) there is scientific evidence to show that a healthy person is one who can play. People who do not have the ability to play or the willingness to play reveal questionable mental health. It is well documented that children who are depressed, have been traumatized, or those with autism have never learned to play (Alvarez and Philips, 1998).

Play is fundamental for children; they build self-esteem and master skills during play activities (White, 1960, 1966; Piaget and Inhelder, 1969; Schaeffer, 1980; Gil, 1991; Erikson, 1963; Nickerson, 1973). Further, Bruner (1986) posits that play is where children can be themselves and interact safely within their environments. This premise evidences that play can be used to improve children's health and help them develop into productive human beings.

Play also is valuable for use with adolescents (Nickerson and O'Laughlin, 1983). With teenagers, play centers around games, such as baseball, basketball, or volleyball. The involvement of motor skills gives adolescents a sense of well-being and mastery and enables them to interact as a team. Bacon (1984) surmised that the Outward Bound program, helps teenagers experience success by pitting them against themselves and a wilderness experience. In this setting, adolescents identify with others and join together to win against nature. Other games such as tennis, golf, or basketball also help teenagers express emotions and work with others (Vernon, 1989; Teeter, Teeter, and Papai, 1976; Gardner, 1983).

Adult play helps relieve the stress of day-to-day responsibilities (Liebmann, 1986). Albert Ellis (1977) established a number of play activities for adults and uses them as therapeutic interventions to let adults experience their unrealistic fears such as the fear of making a mistake or acting inappropriately in front of others. Adult development stages often dictate the type and amount of play that an adult will experience (Erikson, 1963; Gilligan, 1982).

Play among the elderly often depends on their physical and mental abilities. In nursing homes, games are less strenuous and often limited in scope (Mayers and Griffin, 1990). Bouncing or tossing balls, playing cards or a board game, and historical recall games are the most prevalent for senior adults. Nonetheless, the elderly experience and enjoy play activities that help maintain their health, both physical and mental (Mayers and Griffin, 1990).

Family play is more complicated. To be healthy, family play needs to be achieved in a safe environment (i.e. non-competitive, non-hierarchal, and unrestricted), allowing each member a chance to feel good. Establishing priorities is essential in family play, and Watzlawick (1983), best describes how everyone wins in his synopsis of game theory. Game theory offers two ways for people to interact. The first approach, sum-zero, is when someone has to lose. Non-sum-zero allows everyone to win or lose in a non-competitive and safe environment (Watzlawick, 1983). Families need to incorporate the "win-win" concept into their family culture, so that trust is the cornerstone of their family's health and play is the conduit to better family functioning. Individual losses must be minimized during family interactions to maintain respect and safety in fostering good family health.

The most documented therapeutically demonstrated traditions are about children and play, specifically play therapies. Schaeffer (1980) documented the benefits of play by connecting the psychological and developmental returns for the child. Early researchers investigated the advantages of play and play therapy; for example, the use of play to problem-solve, self-express, facilitate communication, and release feelings (Axline, 1949; Piaget and Inhelder, 1969; Ginott, 1961; Erikson, 1963; Nickerson, 1973; White, 1966; Campbell, 1993; Schaeffer, 1980; Gil, 1991). Their early research led to the use of play therapy as a means to help children who were unable to play because of mental or psychological issues (Freud, 1920; Axiline, 1947; 1967). This therapeutic approach continues even today, providing a relationship that enables the child to develop his or her internal abilities to promote improved health and well-being (Landreth, 1982; Bratten and Landreth, 1995; Glass, 1986; Leblanc and Ritchie, 2001; Elliot and Pumfrey, 1972).

Direct and In-Direct Play Therapy

Over the years, play therapy has evolved into two distinct types, direct and in-direct play therapy. Direct play therapy is more client-centered and nonintrusive (Axline, 1967). Guerney (1980) says that direct play therapy is "actually controlled, always centered on the child and attuned to his/her communication, even the subtle ones." In-direct therapies are lengthier, and the therapist offers the child many different play techniques (e.g. art work, puppetry, re-enactment of traumatic events, and story-telling).

The therapist assumes responsibility for managing activities in sessions when providing direct play therapy (Axline, 1967); the therapist may be very active in direct play therapy and inactive in in-direct play therapy. Since its inception, several play therapy theories have advanced; psychoanalytic, structured, behavioral, group, developmental, and sand tray play therapy are now used. Direct play therapies are shorter in duration and provide specific techniques, often tailored to address the child's particular symptoms (Gil, 1991). Gestalt, Filial, and family therapy also are included in the direct play therapy category. Of particular interest to family-health practice is the Filial Play therapy models.

Filial Play Therapy Models

Filial play therapy employs parents or primary caregivers as therapeutic representatives rather than using a child play therapist. This model developed out of a growing demand for new methods to address early childhood emotional difficulties and to ease parents' financial burdens. Ray and colleagues (2000) surmised that Filial play therapy was ideal for improving the relationships between parents and children and moving toward a healthier relationship. Moustakas (1959) suggested that play therapy sessions occur in the home, especially with very young and relatively normal children.

Filial therapy methods developed by Bernard and Louise Guerney (1964), train parents of young children (in groups of six to eight) to conduct play sessions with their children following a specific format. The original model is to be completed within a six to twelve month time frame. Once trained, parents meet weekly with the therapist to discuss the results of their efforts. Play sessions (between the parents and the child) take place in their home, occur two or more times per week, and are between thirty and forty-five minutes long. The therapy program is divided into stages.

During *Stage one*, the parents or caregivers learn to be more empathic and gain a better understanding of the child's needs. They encourage activities (as defined by the child) within specified and defined safety limits, helping the child to know that his or her needs are understood and accepted. They also help the child accept responsibility for his or her actions. This stage develops during approximately six to eight sessions.

In *Stage two*, the therapy begins with using standard play equipment. The therapist helps the parents or caregivers to accept their child's situation and recognize their own emotional reactions during sessions. This is accomplished with tape recordings or note-taking following each session. The number of sessions depends on the amount of therapeutic work that must be completed by the parents or caregivers.

The *final stage* is when the work is completed and the parents move toward termination with the therapist. Theoretically, the emotionally troubled child can now be helped by the parent or caregiver who clearly defines the play and provides corrective and clear feedback over a period of time. In tandem, a therapist guides the process and provides the same parallel process to the parents (Guerney, 1982)

Landreth (1991) developed, implemented, and evaluated a shorter version (ten weeks) of Guerney's (1964) Filial Therapy Model, one with teaching and communication components. During the ten weeks, parents or caregivers meet with a therapist two hours each week to learn basic child-centered techniques practiced in a 30-minute weekly session. A video-taped session also is conducted to provide feedback to parents. Children who are two to ten years old are included in this model; however, older children and teens can participate with some adaptation of activities (Ray, Bratten, and Brandt, 2000).

Research shows that the Filial therapy model is a proven method to help parents achieve a healthier and happier relationship with their child. Parents or caregivers improve their understanding of the child and his or her needs; accept their child's situation; and reduce their child's behavior problems, alleviating the stress level of the parent (Stover and Guerney, 1967; Landreth and Lobaugh, 1998;

Tew, 1997; Glover, 1996; Chau and Landreth, 1997; Bratten, 1993; Bratten and Landreth, 1995).

Other studies, using various populations, point to higher self-esteem for the parent and child (Glass, 1986; Lobaugh, 1991). Filial therapy has been used with single parents (Bratten, 1993; Ray, et.al., 2000), learning-disabled children (Guerney, 1983; Kale, 1997), physically ill children (Glazer-Waldman, 1991; Tew, 1997), children with emotional problems (Sensue, 1981), Native Americans (Glover, 1996), incarcerated mothers (Harris, 1995), incarcerated fathers (Landreth and Lobaugh, 1998), non-offending parents of sexually abused children (Costas and Landreth, 1999), Chinese children and parents (Chau and Landreth, 1997), and mentally disabled children and parents (Boll, 1972). The results of these studies evidence a healthier well-being for the parent and child and incorporate findings of greater parental acceptance, high self-esteem for child and parent, less stress for parent, and improved behavior of the child. The results conclude that human interactions embrace the functions of families within the Family Health model and show that Filial therapy promotes family health practice principles.

Conclusion

As discussed earlier, Family Health focuses on all aspects of the family (e.g. economic, social, physical, emotional, etc.) Individuals within families affect the health issues of each family member and all family members are positively or negatively affected by another member's health status. Effective play enhances all areas of well-being and is connected to all features of the Family Health Model. Filial play therapy helps families use non-sum-zero play to improve family interactions and enable healthy family functions. Families who use Filial play therapy improve their individual and collective well-being. This form of family play helps to establish better communication and understanding and enhances the parent and child relationship (Guerney, 1983; Guerney and Guerney, 1989; Guerney, 1980; Landreth, 1991).

In keeping with the non-sum-zero principle, all family members increase self-esteem and mastery of the skills needed to interact in a healthier manner, promoting all function areas in the Family Health Model. The three function areas most observed and researched that are enhanced by Filial play therapy are the potential for mental growth and development, emotional nurturance, and socialization of family members. Family members who use Filial play therapy, with its non-zero-sum interaction style, are more likely to promote the Family Health Model functions, increasing overall health for all members. Since all areas of family health practice are enhanced by the use of Filial play therapy, this model provides a healthier way to teach appropriate family interactions, change family culture, and promote well-being for all members.

References

Akamatsu, J.T., Hobfoll, S.E., Crowther, J.H. & Stephens, A. (Eds.). (1992). *Family health psychology*. New York: Taylor & Francis.

Alvarez, A. & Phillips, A. (1998). The importance of play: A child psychotherapist's view. *Child Psychology & Psychiatry Review, 3*(3), 99-109.

Axline, V. (1947). *Play therapy: The inner dynamics of childhood.* Cambridge, MA: Houghton-Mifflin.

Axline, V. (1949). Play therapy: A way of understanding and helping reading problems. *Childhood Education, 26*, 156-161.

Axline, V. (1967). *Dibs in search of self.* New York: Ballantine.

Bacon, S. (1984). *The conscious use of metaphor in Outward Bound.* Denver: Colorado Outward Bound School.

Boll, L. (1972) Effects of filial therapy on maternal perceptions of their mentally retarded children's social behavior. Doctoral dissertation, The University of Oklahoma. *Dissertation Abstracts International, 33*, 6661A.

Bratten, S. (1993). Filial therapy with single parents, unpublished doctoral dissertation, University of North Texas, Denton.

Bratten, S., & Landreth, G. (1995). Filial therapy with single parents. *International Journal of Play Therapy, 4*(1), 61-80.

Bruner, J. (1986). Play, thought, and language. *Prospects: Quarterly Review of Education, 16*, 77-83.

Campbell, C. (1993). Play: The fabric of elementary school counseling programs.

Elementary School Guidance & Counseling, 28, 10-16.

Chau, I. & Landreth, G.L. (1997). Filial therapy with Chinese parents: Effects on parental empathic interactions, parental acceptance of child and parental stress. *International Journal of Play Therapy, 6*(2), 75-92.

Cheal, D. (1993). Unity and difference in postmodern families. *Journal of Family Issues, 14*, 5-19.

Costas, M. & Landreth, G. (1999). Filial therapy with non-offending parents of children who have been sexually abused. *International Journal of Play Therapy, 8*(1), 43-66.

Elliott, C., & Pumfrey, P. (1972). The effects of non-directive play therapy on some maladjusted boys. *Educational Research, 14*, 157-163.

Ellis, A. (1977). Fun as psychotherapy. In A. Ellis & R. Grieger (Eds.), *Handbook of rational-emotive therapy* (pp. 262-270). New York: Springer.

Erikson, E.H. (1950). *Childhood and society*. New York: Norton.

Erikson, E.H. (1963). *Childhood and society* (2nd ed.). New York: Norton.

Freud, S. (1920). *Beyond the pleasure principle*. New York: Liverwright.

Gardner, R.A. (1983). The talking, feeling, and doing game. In C.E. Schaefer & K.J. O'Connor (Eds.), *Handbook of play therapy* (pp. 259-273). New York: Wiley.

Gil, E. (1991). *The healing power of play: Working with abused children*. New York: The Guilford Press.

Gilligan, C. (1982). *In a different voice: Psychological theory and women's development*. Cambridge, MA: Harvard University Press.

Ginott, H.G. (1961). *Group psychotherapy with children*. New York: McGraw-Hill.

Glass, N.M. (1986). Parents as therapeutic agents: A study of the effect of filial therapy. Doctoral Dissertation, University of North Texas. *Dissertation Abstracts International, 47*(7), A2457.

Glazer-Waldman, H.R. (1991). *Filial therapy: CPR Training for families with*

chronically ill children. Unpublished master's thesis, University of North
Texas, Denton.

Glover, G.J. (1996). *Filial therapy with Native Americans on the Flathead
Reservation.* Unpublished doctoral dissertation, University of North
Texas, Denton.

Guerney, B. (1964). Filial therapy: Description and rationale. *Journal of
Consulting Psychology, 28,* 303-310.

Guerney, L.G. (1980). Client-centered (nondirective) play therapy. In C. Schaefer
& K. O'Connor (Eds.). *Handbook of play therapy* (pp. 21-64). New York:
Wiley.

Guerney, B. (1982). Filial therapy: Description and rationale. In G.L. Landreth
(Ed.), *Play therapy* (pp. 342-353). Springfield, IL: Thomas.

Guerney, B. & Guerney, L. (1989). Child relationship enhancement: Family
therapy and parent
education. Special issue: Person-centered approaches with families.
*Person Centered
Review, 4,* 344-357.

Guerney, L. (1983). Play therapy with learning disabled children. In C. Schaefer
& K. O'Connor (Eds.), *Handbook of play therapy* (pp. 419-435). New
York: Wiley.

Harris, Z.L. (1995). Filial therapy with incarcerated mothers: A five week model.
International Journal of Play Therapy, 6(2), 53-73.

Kale, A. (1997). *Filial therapy with parents of children experiencing learning
disabilities.* Unpublished doctoral dissertation, University of North Texas,
Denton.

Kochanska, G. (1990). Maternal beliefs as long-term predictors of mother-child
interaction and rapport. *Child Development, 61,* 1934-1943.

Landreth, G. (Ed.). (1982). *Play therapy: Dynamics of the process of counseling
with children.* Springfield, IL: Thomas.

Landreth, G. (1991). *Play therapy: The art of the relationship.* Muncie, IN:
Accelerated Development.

Landreth, G.L. (1993). Child-Centered play therapy. *Elementary School Guidance & Counseling, 28(*1), 17-30.

Landreth, G.L. & Lobaugh, A.F. (1998). Filial therapy with incarcerated fathers: Effects on parental acceptance of child, parental stress, and child adjustment. *Journal of Counseling and Development, 6,*157-165.

Leblanc, M. & Ritchie, M. (2001). A meta-analysis of play therapy outcomes. *Counseling Psychology Quarterly, 14*(1), 149-164.

Liebmann, M. (1986). *Art therapy for groups.* Cambridge, MA: Brookline.

Mayers, K. & Griffin, M. (1990). The play projects: Use of stimulus objects with demented patients. *Journal of Gerontological Nursing, 16,* 32-37.

Mead, G.H. (1934). *Mind, self, and society from the standpoint of a social behaviorist.* Chicago: University of Chicago Press.

Menninger, W. (2003). On play. (as printed in) Menninger Perspective, *33 (3),* p.16). Editor: Roger Verdon.

Moustakas, C.E.(1951). Situational play therapy with normal children. *Journal of Consulting Psychology, 15,* 225-230.

Nickerson, E.T. (1973). Psychology of play and play therapy in classroom activities. *Education Children, Spring,* 1-6.

Nickerson, E.T., & O'Laughlin, K.S. (1983). The therapeutic use of games. In C.E. Schaefer & K.J. O'Connor (Eds*). Handbook of play therapy* (pp. 174-187). New York: Wiley.

Pardeck, J.T., & Yuen, F.K.O. (Eds.) (1999). *Family health: A holistic approach to social work practice.* Westport, CT: Auburn House.

Pardeck, J.T., Yuen, F.K., Daley, J., & Hawkins, K. (1998). Social work assessment and intervention through family health practice. *Family Therapy, 25*(1), 25-39.

Pardeck, J.T., & Yuen, F.K. (2001). Family health: An emerging paradigm for social workers. *Journal of Health and Social Policy, 13*(3), 59-74.

Peterson, G.W., & Rollins, B.C. (1987). Parent-child socialization. In M.B. Sussman & S.K. Steinmetz (Eds.), *Handbook of marriage and family* (pp. 471-507). New York: Plenum.

Piaget, J. (1951). *Play, dreams, and imitation in childhood.* New York: Norton.

Piaget, J. & Inhelder, B. (1969). *The psychology of the child.* (H. Weaver, Trans.). New York: Basic Books.

Ray, D., Bratton, S., & Brandt, M. (2000). Filial/family play therapy for single parents of young children attending community colleges. *Community College Journal of Research & Practice, 24*(6), 469-487.

Schaefer, C.E. (1980). Play therapy. In CG.P. Sholevar, R.M. Benson, & B. J. Blinder (Eds.), *Emotional disorders in children and adolescents.* New York: Spectrum.

Schaefer, C.E. (Ed.) (1993). *The therapeutic powers of play.* Northvale, NJ: Aronson.

Sensue, M.E. (1981). Filial therapy as a potential primary preventative process with children between the ages of four and ten. Doctoral dissertation, The Pennsylvania State University. Dissertation Abstracts International, *42*(01), A148.

Stover, L., & Guerney, B. (1967). The efficacy of training procedures for mothers in filial therapy. *Psychotherapy: Theory, Research, and Practice, 4*(3), 110-115.

Teeter, R., Teeter, T. & Papai, J. (1976). Frustration-A game. *The School Counselor, 23,* 264-270.

Tew, K (1997). *The efficacy of filial therapy with families of chronically ill children.* Unpublished doctoral dissertation, University of North Texas, Denton.

Thornton, M.C., Chatters, L.M., Taylor, R.J., & Allen, W.R. (1990). Sociodemographic and environmental correlates of racial socialization by black parents. *Child Development, 61,* 401-409.

Vernon, A. (1989). *Thinking, feeling, and behaving: An emotional education curriculum for children (grades 7-12).* Champaign, IL: Research.

Watzlawick, P. (1983). *The situation is hopeless, but not serious.* New York: Norton.

White, R. (1960). Competence and the psychosexual stages of development. In

M.R. Jones (ed.). *Nebraska symposium on motivation* (pp. 97-141). Lincoln, NE: University of Nebraska.

White, R. (1966). Lives in progress (2nd ed.). New York: Holt, Rinehart, & Winston.

Wisendale, S.K. (1992). Toward the 21st century: Family change and public policy. *Family Relations, 41,* 417-422.

Zimmerman, S.L. (1992). Family trends: What implications for family policy? *Family Relations, 41,* 423-429.

Chapter 8
Public Health Services to Families: Best Practice
Approaches for Children and Adolescent Well-Being
Harrison Y. Smith

The future of America relies heavily on the health and well-being of the most vulnerable and at-risk population in our society: children and adolescents. Without proper healthcare through careful and persistent early interventions, children and adolescents *cannot, and will not* flourish and become the ideal productive citizens that parents hope and dream they can be.

This chapter will discuss the nature and scope of public health services to families and children, providing information regarding historically evolving structural and health-service contexts. Core functions and essential services are described in relation to public health's impact on families with children. The chapter progresses with a description of the Maternal and Child Health Program, a federally funded initiative with immense resources. This program serves as a broad safety net to ensure that early interventive basic healthcare is provided to low-income families with children. The author identifies and discusses best public-health practices that are rendered by public and private health-care givers.

The case is made for addressing issues of adolescent health care as a critical transitional life-span challenge, followed by a discussion of best practices for assuring optimum healthcare services. Finally, the author discusses ways in which public health practitioners can increase their existing knowledge and skills to include cultural and linguistic competence as a method to improve and facilitate effective public health services to families with children.

The Nature and Scope of Public Health Services to Families with Children

Health service provisions in the United States are generally divided into four categories: physicians and health-related professions that are in private practice, public and private outpatient medical programs, inpatient hospital medical care, and public health services that are funded by tax dollars. Except for broad-scale immunizations, the bulk of day-to-day public health services are ordinarily utilized by individuals, groups, and communities that are not in a socioeconomic status that is privileged. The focus of public health services is primarily preventive with an overarching objective of alleviating large-scale disease epidemics and environmental hazards and providing population-based illness prevention.

Public health services are provided by local municipalities through their health departments, often having strategically decentralized satellite clinics. Many public health services are also provided through government subcontracting through private human service agencies. Services include (not an exclusive list) disease prevention and control; skilled nursing; social work; nutrition; immunizations; school health services; health counseling and family planning; environmental, food, water sanitation, and code enforcement; maintenance and issuance of all birth, death, and marriage certificates, indexing and record-keeping of current communicable diseases; health education; and maternal and child health programs.

Core Functions of Public Health: Transcendence into the 21st Century

Realizing the anachronisms of nineteenth and early twentieth century foci of myopic practices, public health professionals and political influentials began to yield to public demands for embracing social-environmental comprehensive public-health services. Public health began to transcend primary emphasis on infectious diseases and the age of bacteriology, and focused on identifying environmental, behavioral, and social risk factors for chronic diseases and

118

developed *population-based prevention and treatment* methods to reduce these risk factors (Lasker, R. D. and the Committee on Medicine and Public Health, 1997).

As with all human service organizations, public health eventually evolved into a modern and more socially relevant institution. Finally, the Institute of Medicine (1988) and a work group composed of representatives from every conceivable professional health organization, institution, and academia (National Association of County Health Officials, 1994) developed consensus on a list of *core functions and essential services* of public health. Due to public and political pressure, public health was forced to reassess its mission and purpose. It was very important for all public health institutional domains begin to agree on a unitary mission and speak with a single voice. The core functions of public health began to come into fruition.

Core functions of public health as adopted by major institutional domains identified three dimensions, plus a delineated list of (Essential Services Work Group, 1994). Core functions include *assessment* (routine collection, analysis, and sharing information regarding health conditions, risks, and community resources), *policy development* (collecting data, assessment, and development of health and welfare policies and programs for health care delivery), and *assurance* (stressed emphasis on availability of broad-based health services, including coordination and functional operations between public and private providers, demonstrating capacity to respond to critical situations and emergencies.)

Essential services must include health status monitoring, diagnostic and investigatory functions, education and citizen empowerment, developing and mobilizing community partnerships, policy, plans, and program development, code and law enforcement of public-health standards. Linkage, access, and availability of services must be assured as must a competent public health workforce program evaluation effectiveness and ongoing solution-focused health research and program development.

Given this country's history of being bound by a primarily two-party political system and historical roots that are embedded in profit-driven capitalism and the puritan work ethic, the core functions of public health service have not become a reality to the point of reaching the majority of families with children. This is particularly a challenge for families who are near or below the poverty line.

As one of the leading industrialized nations, the United States seriously lags in its attempts to provide adequate health services to families and children. Canada, Japan, and most European countries far excel in health-care provisions to families. The nature and substance of these provisions are comprehensive and wide-ranging, regardless of ability to pay. Life expectancy is highly correlated with the quality of health care in a society. Many industrialized countries with better healthcare systems have a higher life expectancy than the United States (Kornblum and Julian, 2001). How is America responding to the current health-care crisis?

Healthy People 2010 (U. S. Department of Health and Human Services, 2001) is a bold set of health initiatives that have given this nation the impetus and challenge to improve the quality of life for all citizens. It is a comprehensive and dynamic vision with sound health objectives to be accomplished over the first decade of the new century. Inherent in this initiative are two overarching goals that are germane to the health and well-being of children and adolescents who, among others, are more vulnerable and susceptible to unhealthy states. These goals are to increase quality of years of health life and to eliminate health disparities among citizens.

Children and adolescents make up an inordinate number of cases that are reported daily. Cases involve murder, rape, incest, neglect and abuse, suicide, physical and mental illness, homicide, and a variety of unexpected health-related maladies that are antithetical to the maintenance of good health (Guetzloe, 1999). Lower socio-economic families with children are particularly in jeopardy for lacking basic healthcare, vis-à-vis, adequate health insurance coverage. Health insurance coverage is an important component in the maintenance of good health (Paulin and Deitz, 1995).

120

It has been estimated that more than 11 million children, or one in seven, are uninsured in the United States. Declines in employer benefits and increased enrollment in Medicaid insurance (more than 3 million children eligible for Medicaid are not enrolled) are major indicators that the masses of America's children are increasingly experiencing greater health risks (Robert Wood Johnson, 1998).

Insurance eligibility under the 1997 State Children's Health Insurance Program (SCHIP) has been utilized substantially to augment existing public health coverage. This health- care entitlement has been particularly critical to states whose citizens who are known to be disproportionately represented with lower socioeconomic under and unemployed families with children. Under SCHIP one study found that states with higher proportions of low-income uninsured children had greater increases in income eligibility thresholds (Ullman and Hill, 2001).

Public health human service professionals should become demonstrably competent in their comprehension and application of federal healthcare entitlements, particularly when serving disenfranchised low-income families with children. Exhibit 1 delineates the basic features of Medicaid and SCHIP.

EXHIBIT 8.1 – Federal Health Care Programs that Include Child and Adolescent Entitlements (Adapted from Blau and Abramovitz 2004)

Analytical Questions	Health Programs
Medicaid, 1965	
Number of recipients?	36 million.
Who offers the benefit or service?	The states, under federal guidelines.
What form does it take?	Medical coverage.
To whom is it provided?	Low-income people, including the aged, blind, disabled and members of families with dependent children.
At whose expense?	From 50 to 83 % of each state's Medicaid budget comes

	from the federal government's general tax revenue; the states absorb the rest. In 2001, total costs for the Medicaid program amounted to $199 billion.

State Children's Health Insurance program (SCHIP), 1997	
Number of recipients?	4.7 million children were enrolled in SCHIP at some time during 2001.
Who offers the benefit or service?	The states.
What form does it take?	Medical coverage.
To whom is it provided?	Children in families with income up to 200 % of the poverty line.
At whose expense?	$4 billion a year has been allocated for SCHIP's, with the states paying 70 % of the share they assume for Medicaid and the federal government picking up the rest. The revenue comes from an increase in the tobacco tax.

Children and adolescents with chronic health conditions are often overlooked in the scheme of national and local health policy planning. One study (Thies and McAllister, 2001) concluded an estimated 40% of children and adolescents with chronic health conditions experience school-related problems. These authors determined that, unlike their peers with developmental disabilities, students with chronic health conditions do not have the privilege of accessing special education service programs. The chronically unhealthy child and adolescent population (especially in poor urban and rural areas) are continuously in need of regular education with special circumstances, while simultaneously having the same degree of need for accommodations to address their unique health conditions.

Under similar circumstances, studies have shown that families of children with chronic conditions, who are on welfare, indicate minimal knowledge and awareness of policies affecting their *continued eligibility and maintenance* of services when the child's illness may cause employment disruption (Smith, Wise, and Wampler, 2002). This issue is critical inasmuch as receiving Temporary Assistance for Needy Families' (TANF) benefits are subject to termination if work requirements are not followed. Knowledge of work requirements, time limits, time limit extensions and applications for exemptions and extensions are often ignored, placing the family and children with chronic illnesses in grave harm.

Maternal and Child Health: The Genesis Formula as Predictor for Positive Child and Adolescent Life-Span Development

It is virtually impossible to expect and succeed in acquiring optimum biopsychosocial health through life-span development without understanding and engaging in healthy behaviors from birth to the end of one's life. Families, communities, and public health officials have known this simple fact since the beginning of America as a nation. Although early social thought embraced a combination of religion and science to provide health-care services, phenomena of wars, social experiments, experiences from catastrophic events, and modern scientific developments have had strong influences on congress to evolve and address issues of public health.

The United States Congress has passed a plethora of laws to ensure that multiple health care safety networks are in place and functional for the health and well-being of families. For example:

- Title XIX of the Social Security Act authorized Medicaid;
- Title X of the Public Health Services Act sanctioned Family Planning and Population Research;
- Title IV of the Personal Responsibility and Work Opportunity Reconciliation Act transformed AFDC into Temporary Assistance to Needy Families;
- Title XXI of the Social Security Act (State Children's Health Insurance Plan) subsidized states to provide basic medical insurance to low-income children;

123

- and Title V of the Social Security Act (Maternal and Child Health, Children With Special Health Care Needs) funds programs to assure sustained improvement in health, safety, and well-being of mothers, prenatal, postnatal, child, and adolescents.

Implementation of the Maternal and Child Health legislation was a visionary, compassionate, and progressive action toward assurance of creating positive early child and adolescent life-span development for low-income families. Good prenatal care reduces the incidence of low birth weight. Mothers who do not receive prenatal care are three to five times more likely to have low-birth-weight babies than mothers who receive this care in the first trimester (Gilbert, E. S. and Harmon, J. S., 1986; McDonald, T. P. and Coburn, A. F., 1988; Pierson, V. H. et al, 1994). Birth weight is critical to health maintenance because low-birth-weight infants are 40 times more likely to die during their first month than normal weight infants.

Visionary compassionate progressiveness notwithstanding, needy low-income families continue to be discovered without adequate nutrition and health services, especially in the area of prenatal care. In many cases, existing access barriers are formidable. For example, mothers are at high risk for not having transportation to make appointments and for having health-care system intrapersonal issues and inadequacy of prenatal care that poses grave risks to both mother and child (Cook, et al, 1999). Late entry into prenatal care, owing to distressed urban neighborhood context, and managed-care restrictions are also major health deterrents. (Perloff and Jaffee (1999).

The Institute of Medicine's Committee to Study the Prevention of Low Birth Weight (1985) identified six barriers to obtaining effective prenatal care:

- Lack of insurance or inadequate insurance
- Lack of maternity care providers for low-income high-risk women.
- Inadequate prenatal services in the clinical sites where high-risk women utilize.
- Beliefs, attitudes, and experiences among women which discourage accessing prenatal care.

- Lack of transportation and child care services.
- Inadequate facilities/systems to provide care for hard-to-reach women.

Economy of scale, when applied sensibly, and with smart marketing strategies, can stimulate and influence reluctant families with children to maximize greater use of available maternal and child health services. For example, better education about nutrition is critically important to the health and well-being of both mother and child. Old habits about nutrition may be one of the most lethal weapons that contribute to low birth weight and deterring healthy longevity.

The American Public Health Association's (APHA) Governing Council has recently adopted a policy that focuses on food marketing, children and overweight (The Nations Health, 2003). Their policy encourages measures to ban food advertising from schools, supports school policies that promote healthy eating environments, advocates for legislation banning food advertising during children's television programs, and advocates development of guidelines that demonstrate responsible food advertising and marketing.

APHA has also adopted a policy that advocates additional funding for women and children that encourages breastfeeding, healthy eating and physical activity. The policy calls for full funding of the Special Supplemental Nutrition Program for Women, Infants, and Children (WIC program); increased fruit and vegetable intake through school lunch programs; and increased access to child-nutrition programs by eliminating the reduced price-category.

Many health and human service professionals are unaware of existing public and privately sponsored food programs, number of recipients, forms of delivery, and how these programs are funded. From a "best-practice" perspective, health care case managers, concerned with quality of service delivery, should be informed, and educate consumers about these programs. Exhibit 2 identifies and briefly describes the most- utilized food programs that are available to low-income families. Readers are especially encouraged to review the Special Supplemental Nutrition Program for Women, Infants, and Children. It is more popularly known as the WIC Program. It was designed to ensure the health of low-income women, infants, and children up to five years of age who are at nutritional risk. The program provides nutritious foods to supplement diets, information on health eating, and referrals to health-care providers.

EXHIBIT 8.2 – Federally-Sponsored Food Programs for Families, Children, and Adolescents (Adapted from Blau and Abramovitz, 2004)

Analytical Questions	FOOD PROGRAMS
Food Stamps (Bridge Card) 1964	
Number of recipients?	19.3 million people (2002).
Who offers the benefit or service?	The state and local government are primarily responsible of the day-to-day administration of the program.
What form does it take?	A voucher for food.
To whom is it provided?	Households with gross incomes below 130 % of the poverty line, which means that most TANF, SSI and general assistance recipients are automatically eligible.
At whose expense?	The federal government assumes responsibility for the cost of all food stamp benefits and half of the state's administrative costs. In 2001, total federal expenditures reached $17.5 billion.
Special Supplemental Nutrition Program for Women, Infants, and Children (WIC), 1972	
Number of recipients?	7.5 million people.
Who offers the benefit or service?	The federal government.
What form does it take?	A voucher for specific foods.
To whom is it provided?	Pregnant women, new mothers, infants, and children up to 5 years of age with income less than 185 % of the poverty line.
At whose expense	The federal government pays for the total cost, which is currently budgeted at about $4.4 billion annually.
National School Lunch Program, 1946	
Number of recipients?	27 million children.
Who offers the benefit or	98,000 public and private nonprofit elementary and

service?	secondary schools and residential child care institutions.
What form does it take?	Lunch at free or reduced prices.
To whom is it provided?	School children from families with gross income below 130 % of the poverty line receive lunch for free; those between 130 and 185 % of the poverty line receive reduced-price lunches.
At whose expense?	The federal government pays for the program, which costs about $5.556 billion

National School Breakfast, 1966

Number of recipients?	7.9 million children.
Who offers the benefit or service?	72,000 schools and residential centers.
What form does it take?	Free or reduced-price breakfasts.
To whom is it provided?	School children from families with gross income below 130 % of the poverty line receive lunch for free; those between 130 and 185 % of the poverty line receive reduced-price lunches.
At whose expense?	The federal government pays for the program, which cost $1.49 billion in 2001.

Summer Food Services, 1968

Number of recipients?	2.1 million children, plus 1.1 million for lunches.
Who offers the benefit or service?	Public and private nonprofit institutions.
What form does it take?	Free or reduced-price summer breakfasts and lunches.
To whom is it provided?	School children, according to the same eligibility standards as in the National School Breakfast and Lunches Program. Schoolchildren, according to the same eligibility standards as in the National School Lunch programs.
At whose expense?	The federal government, at a cost of $298 million.

Child and Adult care Food program (CACFP), 1968	
Number of recipients?	2.5 million children and 67,000 elderly daily.
Who offers the benefit or service?	Day-care centers, private non-profit adult day-care facilities, homeless shelters, Head start and after school programs
What form does it take?	Free or reduced-price meals and snacks.
To whom is it provided?	Children, according to the same eligibility standards as in the National School Breakfast and National School Lunch programs, and adults who are either functionally impaired over age 60.
At whose expense?	The federal government relies on grants to the states to pay for CACFP. The states then distribute this money to local social agencies. In 2000, the program's budget was $1.6 billion.
The Emergency Food Assistance Program	
Number of recipients?	4 million households annually.
Who offers the benefit or service?	The emergency food assistance network: community kitchens and food banks.
What form does it take?	Surplus commodities.
To whom is it provided?	Poor people who meet state guidelines that determine eligibility for surplus food.
At whose expense?	The federal government spends about $200 million annually on TEFAP.
Private Food Assistance Network (early 1980s)	
Number of recipients?	At least 23 million people annually (the number served by Second Harvest, one of its umbrella organizations)
Who offers the benefit or service?	Community kitchens and food pantries.
What form does it take?	More than 2 billion pounds annually.
To whom is it provided?	Poor people who cannot afford to pay the market price for food.
At whose expense?	Everyone who donates food or money to a food charity.

Best Public Health Practices for Maternal and Child Health

Although governmental stewardship is often perceived as stingy with resources for low-income families, best practices for intervention exist and are in place. Assuming public health units of government and contracting private health providers are able to navigate these barriers, Friedenberg and Grason (1997) identified and delineated "10 essential public health services" to promote maternal and child health in America. Public health physicians, social workers, nurses, and other allied-health professionals and their institutions are duty-bound to provide families with children the following essential public health services:

- Access and monitor maternal and child health status and resolve needs.
- Diagnose and investigate health problems and hazards.
- Inform and educate the public and families about maternal and child health issues.
- Mobilize community partnerships between policy makers, health care providers, families, general public, and others to identify and solve maternal and child health problems.
- Provide leadership for priority-setting, planning, and policy development to support community efforts to assure the health of women, children, and families.
- Promote and enforce legal requirements that protect the health and safety of women, children, and ensure public accountability for their well-being.
- Link women and children to health and other community and family services, and assure access to comprehensive, quality health care systems.
- Assure capacity and competency of the public health and personal heal health workforce to effectively address maternal and child health needs.
- Evaluate the effectiveness, accessibility, and quality of personal health and population-based maternal and child health services.
- Support research and demonstrations to gain new insights and innovative solutions to maternal and child health-related problems.

Both overarching and underlying criteria for use of best practice capacity and competency of health professionals are demonstration of a thorough knowledge foundation base of risk and opportunity factors that influence the level of quality of maternal and child health care. For example, treatment expertise notwithstanding, it is crucial for practitioners to understand the basic levels of primary prevention (focus on preventing disease or condition from occurring; health promotion and protection) secondary prevention (early diagnosis and treatment; focus on delaying or averting conditions after onset); and tertiary prevention (preventing further disability and deterioration; focus on rehabilitation and or restoring clients to improved functioning upon full onset of disease or condition.).

Professional knowledge foundation also includes acute awareness and understanding behavioral and structural determinants that affect the ultimate outcome of mothers and children's health. For example, poor nutrition, smoking, substance use and abuse, stress, age, race, gender, class, education, and environmental hazards may heavily influence the outcome of maternal and child health. Just as important is the demand for health-care providers and practitioners to give the highest priority to *Early and Periodic Screening, Diagnosis and Treatment* (EPSDT). This means educating and advocating for families to ensure that their children have access to and engage in regular periodic medical, vision, hearing, and dental screenings.

The Case for Improving and Sustaining Adolescent Health

Adolescence is a period of intense change, characterized by multiple biopsychosocial significant life-changing transitions on a tenuous path toward healthy development. Immediate and extended families, fictive kin, and larger environments often fall short in the provision of strong social supportive networks that are necessary for adolescents to make rational and responsible decisions about health development. Consequently, adolescents are constantly challenged to assure that risky health behaviors are minimized.

Although not totally inclusive, aversive risk factors that preclude optimum adolescent health include peer pressure, substance abuse, sexually transmitted infectious diseases, pregnancy, unintentional injury, healthcare access, age, race, gender, and class. Early interventions are critical not only to ensure physical health but also to provide quality mental health services to a population that is more susceptible to psychological challenges due to rapid growth identity development transitions and the importance of peers.

Best Public Health Practices for Optimum Adolescent Development

According to Klein et al. (1992), public health service providers should demonstrate a basic level of professional competence across disciplines regarding adolescent health delivery. Minimally, adolescents should always voice satisfaction with the quality of health care received. Health services should be convenient and visible; access should not require extensive planning by either adolescents or their families.

Proactive outreach programs should be in place to educate adolescents and their families, both in use and about the importance of health prevention. One study suggests the strong need for parents to be informed on the ways in which they can best rear their children for maximum competence so that these children and adolescents might reach their highest levels of well-being (Slicker and Thornberry, 2003). Issues of confidentiality should be resolved in the best interest and to the satisfaction of the adolescent consumer.

The cost of health care is always of grave concern, especially to families with less than adequate financial resources to procure services from private health-care institutions. Poverty is affirmed to be the most critical factor affecting and influencing adolescent health (Klien, et al, 1992). Affordability of health care for all children and adolescents should be mandated by federal and state legislation. Insurance programs such as SCHIP, Medicaid, and employer group insurance plans should include preventive services, allowing adequate time and substance to meet adolescent-specific health care needs.

Vulnerable at-risk populations should receive the utmost attention and parity with mainstream citizens whose access to health care systems is more readily available. Cultural, ethnic, and social diversity should receive maximum attention and consideration during health policy planning and program implementation. All health plans should give priority to the transition between pediatric and adult health care.

Overall, adolescent health care should avoid the pitfalls of fragmented services as well as being subjected to "conveyer-belt medicine." That is, health care services should always include the highest level of comprehensiveness that encapsulates mental, medical, and psychosocial services. Correspondingly, adolescent health care should be given with substantive duration to avoid the existing prevalence of low-quality time-limited services that is provided in deference to the imposing demands of managed-care systems.

Family-Centered Practice in Public Health: Improving Cultural and Linguistic Competence in Response to Diversity in Families with Children

Culturally and linguistically responsiveness to consumers in need of human services is a serious challenge regardless of context. Contemporary American society is fraught with complexity, requiring enormous energy and intellect to achieve basic survival and beyond. The world that we have is the one that we have created. We are a product of critical traditions interpreted by and through media of sociologists, economists, historians, and politicians. Our scholarship has created a myth-laden set of social institutions, requiring the need to demythologize the *ideal images* of the American family and re-examine the diversity of contemporary families that will draw us closer to reality (Zinn and Eitzen, 2002).

The challenge of providing cultural and linguistically competent public health services requires new commitments, vigilance, honesty, and ethnocentric desensitization. From a public health perspective, the rationales for addressing these issues enables health-care institutions to effectively respond to demographic changes, and improve health care quality and outcomes (Campinha-Bacote, 2002). The discussion that follows focuses on recommendations for achieving a basic understanding and skill level for bridging cultural and linguistic gaps to enhance public health services to children, adolescents, and their families.

Family-Centered Early Interventions

Inasmuch as life span development is a growth continuum, it is important to emphasize *early intervention* programs (medical and psychosocial) that have strong credibility. Epps and Jackson (2000) identify five principles that are key to designing and implementing effective interventions with children from birth to five years of age when focusing on developmental challenges or with children who are at-risk for delays.

The first principle is providing services that are *family centered*. This means focusing on the family as active members, involved in need identification and all aspects of service interventions. Such a partnership is built on trust, respect, and open communication. Family-centered services expand through use of natural social supportive networks.

Second, parishioners focus their attention on *competence and resilience* of the child and her/his family, identifying strengths and resilience as critical social capital. Resilience in the child and family can be identified through coping capacities, pro-health adaptiveness, and endurance.

Third, early intervention utilizes an *integrated service delivery system* through community-building processes; it forges family and agency partnerships. This is an empowering process as family members are embraced as a vital part of the decision-making process of needs-meeting. Agency professionals give deference to family members in priority-setting, election of services, and acquiring of ownership.

Fourth, caregivers utilize a *systems approach* to discern the nature of relationships within and external to the family as a means of optimizing and facilitating change in the lives of children and families.

Fifth, and finally, early intervention strategies should be *science-based (empirically driven)*. Authenticity of voice (of child and family), combined with objective analyses and disciplined assessments, should be augmented with existing best practice methodologies that are drawn from valid research findings and applied literature.

Cultural Competence

By definition, cultural competence as a concept has many vagaries. From an integrative micro-mezzo-macro systems perspective, cultural competence may be defined as a set of congruent behaviors, attitudes, and policies that come together in a system, agency, or among professionals and enable that system, agency or those professionals to work effectively in cross-cultural situations (Batts and Campinha, 2002). In other terms, cultural competence transcends race and ethnicity; rather, it encapsulates many social demographic variables.

In direct practice, cultural competence begins with healthcare professionals. It is based on consumer-provider relationships. First-time interaction sets the stage for either a positive or a negative beginning, and will have a lasting impact on the consumer. The following list provides examples of obstacles to culturally competent healthcare (Batts and Campinha-Bacote, 2002).

- Stereotypes, biases and assumptions
- Viewing culture as "them," not me
- Confounding race, culture, and ethnicity
- Differing health belief models
- Patient exploitation and oppression
- Pseudo-explanatory models
- Cultural mismatches
- Language and communication barriers
- Misdiagnosing ethnic-specific medical concerns
- Cultural clashes

In addition to the above obstacles, medical professionals quite often assume a crippling sense of superiority, readily dismissing racial and ethnic-specific medical concerns; falsely assuming the patient is not qualified and/or ignorant of her/his medical condition. Additionally, physicians, physician assistants, and nurses invariably are reluctant to provide thorough, *hands-on* physical examination to people of color, preferring to "talk their way through" an examination. Anecdotally, anonymous cases have been reported to have more difficulty obtaining a physical examination when the physician is a white or Asian female and the patient is a black adult male. Do mothers and children of color have the same experiences? Are these anecdotal experiences representative of the general population? Facts are not readily available.

The Institute of Medicine (2002) has recommended several actions to address healthcare racial and ethnic disparities: (1) increase awareness of these disparities among the general public and key stakeholders; (2) increase healthcare provider's awareness of disparities; (3) initiate legal, regulatory, and policy interventions to enact change; and (4) and develop and implement data collection and monitoring systems to address needs, evaluation effectiveness, and a myriad of other purposes that improves healthcare.

Freeman (2002) proposes building cultural competence to ensure sustained changes in the culture of organizations. The author presents a myriad of strategies: (1) be strategic in approaches to promoting cultural competence (accept few assumptions); (2) build an infrastructure for cultural competence (large change is built on small steps); (3) recognize the importance of people and relationships (work hard at building relationships; minimize conflict); (4) convert failed attempts into positive outcomes; (5) use the management and tools you use for other issues; and (6) increase readiness for change by building internal support for anticipated initiatives.

Assuming children, adolescents, and their families survive issues and experiences owing to ethnic, racial, and cultural differences, increasingly, many families have serious difficulties obtaining much needed linguistic services. This barrier is often enormously formidable, creating critical gaps in the provision of effective public health service delivery. The following section addresses this issue and identifies ways in which children, adolescents, and families with language barriers may have improved access to quality of healthcare.

Linguistic Services: Translation and Interpretation Issues

More often than one would like to believe, language barriers are difficult to overcome by both immigrants and Americans whose regional dialects different from the "King's English." Health-care institutions are increasingly sensitive to this issue but have a long way to go before having in place accommodations to facilitate effective patient-provider interaction. The Western medicine mindset suggests the need to understand the value differences between American medical culture and alternative non-western cultures.

Power differentials between Western medical professionals and patients who come from other ethnic and racial cultures are markedly skewed in favor of the professionals. This difference causes strong reluctance of patients to communicate their medical concerns, and conversely, creates awkwardness in communication on the part of the professional. Both parties are frustrated, causing some level of failure to provide quality of health-care.

The following conundrum depicts the challenge for rendering quality health-care to children, adolescents, and their families from different cultural backgrounds:

> Styles of communication may differ among patients from various cultural backgrounds...beyond language differences. Considering all types of communication (e.g., written, spoken and body language; dialects; and slang) the importance of patient- provider interaction hangs in the balance between good and bad medicine (author interpretation adjusting for syntax). Some communication challenges include medical terminology versus common terms, varying literacy levels, the speed of speech, culturally inappropriate words or phrases, multiple dialects, the use and misuse of interpreters and gender-specific terminology (Batts, 2002, p. 14).

Batts' exhibit demonstrates the following guidelines (adaptation) to suggest ways in which health-care providers may address improving interactions with culturally diverse patients (See Exhibit 3). These guidelines are general in nature, content, and scope and are flexible to change, depending on geographic regions. Health care providers are best equipped to address issues and challenges of linguistic services provisions for families in their culturally diverse communities.

EXHIBIT 8.3 – Suggested Guidelines for Improving Patient-Provider Linguistic Services and Relationships

Basic Concerns	Questions to Help Providers Understand Families and Children
Names	How are people named? Do given or family names come first? Are titles used? Do names change?
History	Why did the family immigrate here? Where from? What are conditions in the home country or local region in the United States? What health conditions exist there? What is the work history of the family?
Language	What language or dialect is spoken? Are there differences in the speaking styles (English proficiency and slings) between parents and siblings?
Religion	What are the spiritual beliefs and do they impact daily routines? Are there any medical taboos? How does religion impact care decisions?
Moral Beliefs	What do patients believe about pregnancy, unwanted pregnancy, sexually transmitted diseases or similar conditions? How does this affect care decisions and disclosure to physicians or other human service professions?
Foods and Beverages	What food and beverages are common? Are there any taboo foods and beverages? What are the social rules concerning food and beverages?
Community	What services are available in the community? Is this a unified or divided community? How does community self-help factor into the lives of residents?
Acculturation	How long has the family/individual resided in the U.S.? To what degree has each individual family member adopted American culture (or the local culture compared to another region of the U.S.)

In addition to issues of access, the availability of appropriate linguistic services is critical to quality and culturally competent healthcare. Linguistic services are divided into four categories of services: oral, interpretation, written, and translation (Batts, 2002). Issues of under-use, propensity for malpractice liability, and federal law violation are but a few concerns that face healthcare providers. The latter issue focuses on the existence of federal laws that mandate health-care providers to ensure language services to all limited English proficiency persons (LEP). These laws include the Hill Burton Hospital Survey Construction Act of 1946, Title VI of the Civil Rights Act of 1964, and the Disadvantaged Minority Health Improvement Act of 1990).

Healthcare providers have multiple options to provide linguistic services to families with children. Though not totally inclusive, the following options are presented as appropriate choices, depending on size, need, and capacity of any given healthcare agency.

- Hiring permanent bilingual and bicultural staff (with collateral agency duties)
- Subcontracting outside interpreters
- Hiring, and having as-needed telephone interpretation services (for emergencies and special case situations)
- Use of video conferencing translation and computer software utilization

Although many health-care agencies rely on English-proficient family members to assist in translation and interpretation, prevailing literature and research suggest that providers should resist this temptation, particularly with children. Many families of different cultures are highly sensitive to patriarchical and matriarchic authority structures where children are viewed as having a subordinate status. Placing a child in a position of having to "step out of their place" may cause serious harm to family relationships.

Discussion

Child and adolescent health care is a serious matter, requiring the highest priority. The nation's future depends on the health and well-being of all children. The amount of expenditures on health care is staggering, but too little is directed toward a very large segment of the nation's child population, especially on low-income families with children. Malnutrition, inadequate pre- and postnatal care, educational deprivation, sexually transmitted diseases, violence, and substance abuse are only a few social problems that challenge the child and adolescent population.

The mission and goals of public health services are laudable. The institution's core functions and essential healthcare services are comprehensive and substantive. Maternal and Child Health Programs provide early interventions that seem to work well. Adolescent healthcare is challenging and needs more extensive surveillance and attention. This is particularly critical to low-income adolescents.

The rapid growth in the number of Americans with minority status, particularly people of color, has caused that group to be the least cared-for. Cultural and linguistic competency is seriously lacking as a means of bridging cultures and enhancing health-care for families with children and adolescents. The primary formula for healthy families and sustained well-being is vigilance, resiliency of the human spirit, political empowerment (emphasis on the importance of voting), the academy (emphasis on quality education), and family values that give the highest priority to the latter parts of the formula.

References

Batts, F. and Campinha-Bacote, J. (May 30, 2002). Cultural competency: The basics. Conference Workshop presentation. *Bridging cultures and enhancing care: Approaches to cultural and linguistic competency in managed care*. Chicago: Conference sponsored by the Health Resources and Service Administration (HRSA), Center for Health Services Financing and Managed Care, and American Public Human Service Association (APHSA).

Blau, J. and Abramovitz (2004). The dynamics of social welfare policy. New York: Oxford University Press.

Blueprint for a health community (1994). Washington, DC: National Association of County Health Officials.

Cook, C. A. L., Selig, K. L., Wedge, B. J., and Gohn-Baube, E. A. (March 1999).

Access barriers and the use of prenatal care by low-income, inner-city women, *Social* Work, *44*(2), 129-139.

Core public health functions: A progress report from the Washington State Core government public health functions task force (January, 1993). Olympia, WA: Washington Department of Health.

Epps, S. and Jackson, B. J. (2000). *Empowered families, successful children: Early intervention programs that work.* Washington, DC: American Psychological Association

Essential Services Work Group (Spring 1994). *Essential services of public health.* Washington, DC: Association of State and Territorial Health Officials, National Association of County and City Health Officials, Institute of Medicine (National Academy of Sciences), Association of Schools of Public Health, Public Health Foundation, National Association of State Alcohol and Drug Abuse Directors, National Association of State Mental Health Program Directors, and Public Health Service.

Freeman, C. (March 30, 2002). Building cultural competence in organizations: Focus on promoting and sustaining change. *Bridging cultures and enhancing care: Approaches to cultural and linguistic competency in managed care.* Chicago: Health Resources and Services Administration, Center for Health Services Financing and Managed Care, and American Public Human Services Association.

Friedenberg, L. A, and Grason, H. (1997). *Public MCH Program Functions Framework: Essential Public Health Services to Promote Maternal and Child Health in America.* Washington, DC: U. S. Department of Health and Human Services. Maternal and Child Health Bureau.

Gilbert, E. S. and Harmon, J. S. (1986). High-risk pregnancy and delivery. St. Louis: C. V. Mosby.

Guetzloe, E. (1999). Violence in children and adolescents-A threat to public health and safety: A paradigm for prevention. *Preventing School Failure, 44*(1), 21-24.

Kornblum, W. and Julian, J. (2001). *Social problems,* 10th ed. Upper Saddle

River, NJ:Prentice Hall.

Lasker, R. D. and the Committee on Medicine and Public Health (1997). New York: The New York Academy of Medicine.

McDonald, T. P. and Coburn, A. F. (1988). Predictors of prenatal care utilization. *Social Science and Medicine, 27*, 167-172.

Paulin, G. D. and Dietz, E. M. (1995). Health insurance coverage for families with children. *Monthly Labor Review, 118*, 13-23.

Perloff, J. D. and Jaffee, K. D. (March 1999). Late entry into prenatal care: The neighborhood context. *Social Work*, 44(20), 118-128.

Pierson, V. H., Schramm, W., Stockbauer, J., Land, G., Hoffman, H., and Herman, A. (1994). Prenatal care access and pregnancy outcomes in Missouri. *Missouri Medicine, 91, 624-629.*

Slicker, E. K. and Thornberry, I. (2003). Older adolescent well-being and authoritative   parenting. *Adolescent and Family Health. 3*(1), 9-19.

Summaries of 2003 Policies Passed by the Governing Council (December 2003). *The Nation's Health.* Washington, DC: American Public Health Association.

The Institute of Medicine (March 2002). *Racial and ethnic disparities in healthcare.* Washington, DC: National Academies.

The Institute of Medicine (National Academies) (June, 1998). *America's children: Health insurance.* Second Report: *Systems of accountability: Implementing children's health insurance programs.* Princeton, NJ: Robert Wood Johnson Foundation.

Thies, K. M. and McAllister, J. W. (May 2001). The health and education leadership   project: A school initiative for children and adolescents with chronic health   conditions. *Journal of School Health, 71*(5), 167-172.

The Institute of Medicine (1988). *The future of public health.* Washington, DC: National Academy Press.

Ullman, F. and Hill, I. (2001). Eligibility under state children's health insurance programs. *American Journal of Public Health, 91*, 1449-1451.

U. S. Department of Health and Human Services. (February, 2001). *Healthy people in   health communities: A community planning guide using healthy people 2010.* Washington, DC: Office of Disease Prevention and Health Promotion.

Chapter 9
Family Health Practice and Chronic Illness Among
Children and Adolescents
John Gunther

Mary Sue Marz

What is Chronic Illness?

Dictionary.com (2003) defines chronic as "of long duration; continuing; lasting for a long period of time or marked by frequent recurrence, as certain diseases," and illness as "poor health resulting from disease of body or mind; sickness." Chronic illness may encompass a protracted course that can be progressive and fatal, or it can be associated with a relatively normal life span despite impaired functioning. Frequently there are periods of acute exacerbations that may require intensive medical and psychosocial attention.

For children and adolescents with a chronic illness, the symptoms do not go away. Pain and lack of energy may be constant. There may be physical changes or decreased functioning that affects appearance, resulting in lowered self-esteem, withdrawal from family, friends, and social activities. Friends and family may need to alter their daily activities and social interactions due to the needs of the child with a chronic illness. For all involved, it becomes a challenge of living with chronic uncertainty.

Chronic Illness and the Family

Faux (1997) notes that advances in health care have improved and prolonged lives of children with chronic illnesses. Chronically ill children and adolescents spend most of their lives in the community, not in a hospital or institution. For maximum quality of life, children with chronic illness is primarily dependent on themselves and their families. The effects of a child with a long-term illness, the care required, and the adjustments that must be made make heavy demands on the family system and may require the family to make permanent sacrifices (Christian, 1993). The chronic illness will influence all aspects of family functioning–the budget, housing, transportation, work practices, amount of time parents spend with siblings, educational plans, and all family dynamics. Parents and siblings may become involved in daily activities such as school participation, medications, special diets, transportation, supervision to prevent injury, and physical therapy. Families may bend, or collapse under these demands. The child becomes the concern of social workers, teachers, psychologists, educational consultants, public and private health agency personnel, clergy, and all others who may be working with them to cope with their chronic illness. Previous work found that understanding the parents' stance provided a foundation for individualizing interventions and interactions of not only the disease but also of the family's experience of the illness.

In addition to understanding the parents' stance and when considering the role of chronic illness with adolescents and children, it is imperative to critically analyze the developmental needs of children and adolescents and the role that family plays in addressing the issues involved that enhance the quality of life for the chronically ill child, and perhaps that best-known developmental theory for psychosocial development is articulated by Erickson (1963). These stages reflect the developmental challenges for the chronically ill child and his/her family. In sum, Erickson's stages are noted below (About.com, 2003).

Stage 1: Infancy -- Age 0–1

Crisis. Trust vs Mistrust

Description. In the first year of life, infants depend on others for food, warmth, and affection, and therefore must be able to blindly trust the parents (or caregivers) for providing those.

Positive Outcome. If their needs are met consistently and responsively by the parents, infants not only will develop a secure attachment with the parents, but will learn to trust their environment in general as well.

Negative Outcome. If these needs are not met, infants will develop mistrust towards people and things in their environment, even towards themselves.

Stage 2: Toddler -- Age 1–2

Crisis. Autonomy (Independence) vs. Doubt (or Shame)

Description. Toddlers learn to walk, talk, use toilets, and do things for themselves. Their self-control and self-confidence begin at this stage.

Positive Outcome. If parents encourage their child's use of initiative and reassure them when they make mistakes, the children will develop the confidence needed to cope with future situations that require choice, control, and independence.

Negative Outcome. If the parents are overprotective, or disapproving of the child's acts of independence, they may begin to feel ashamed of their behavior, or have too much doubt of their abilities.

Stage 3: Early childhood – Age 2–6

Crisis. Initiative vs. Guilt

Description. Children have newfound power at this stage as they have developed motor skills and become more and more engaged in social interaction with people around them. They now must learn to achieve a balance between eagerness for more adventure and more responsibility, and learning to control impulses and childish fantasies.

Positive Outcome. If parents are encouraging, but consistent in discipline, children will learn to accept without guilt, that certain things are not allowed, but at the same time will not feel shame when using their imagination and engaging in make-believe role plays.

Negative Outcome. If not, children may develop a sense of guilt and may come to believe that it is wrong to be independent. Learning to talk about emotions and feelings is important for children's mental health, but it is also challenging.

Stage 4: Elementary and Middle School Years – Age 6–12

Crisis. Competence (aka. "Industry") vs. Inferiority.

Description. School is the important event at this stage. Children learn to make things, use tools, and acquire the skills to be a worker and a potential provider. And they do all these while making the transition from the world of home into the world of peers.

Positive Outcome. If children can discover pleasure in intellectual stimulation, being productive, seeking success, they will develop a sense of competence.

Negative Outcome. If not, they will develop a sense of inferiority.

Stage 5: Adolescence – Age 12–18

Crisis. Identity vs. Role Confusion

Description. This is the time when we ask the question, "Who am I?" To successfully answer this question, Erickson suggests the adolescent must integrate the healthy resolution of all earlier conflicts. Did we develop the basic sense of trust? Do we have a strong sense of independence and competence, and do we feel in control of our lives? Adolescents who have successfully dealt with earlier conflicts are ready for the "Identity Crisis," which is considered by Erickson the single most significant conflict a person must face.

Positive Outcome. If the adolescent solves this conflict successfully, he or she will come out of this stage with a strong identity, and ready to plan for the future.

Negative Outcome. If not, the adolescent will sink into confusion and will be unable to make decisions and choices, especially about vocation, sexual orientation, and her or his role in life in general.

Family Health Practice

As a start for the family health practitioner, an assessment must be conducted as a basis for intervention. It must be understood that a chronic illness should be differentiated from an acute illness because the effects of a chronic illness have substantively more impact on daily functioning. Elements to be considered in a *family health assessment* include the following.

- Determine how the chronic illness affects the physical, social and personal adjustments of the individual's and family life.

- Evaluate whether psychological and family interventions are needed and how they would improve the quality of life for the individual and family. Elements to evaluate include anxiety, depression, interpersonal distress, social isolation, and whether there is a positive adjustment to the chronic illness.

- Evaluate functioning and adjustment to the chronic illness including such factors as the role of siblings, caregivers, mother and father, and the economic means and resources and accessibility support for ongoing health care.

Development

Depending on the specific illness, the severity and effects of a chronic illness may change as the child grows older and as the body goes though normal maturational changes. Especially during adolescence, previously routine treatments may need to be changed both because of the adolescent's changing body and because of the teen's increasing need for independence, responsibility, and privacy. Also changing as the child grows older is the child's understanding of illness: The following developmental cycles by Potter (1998) are illustrative.

Birth to 18 months. Infants do not realize that illness is not a part of normal life. Very young children do not understand that objects and people still exist even when they cannot see them; thus separations from family may be especially painful.

18-36 months. Toddlers understand their illness only as something that interferes with their own world. They have a magical view of causes and effects leading them to believe that if they want something to happen it will happen; or they may believe it was something they thought or did that made them sick. Toddlers also need to feel that they have some control over their world.

3-7 years. Preschoolers are beginning to think more logically but still tend to believe that bad things, such as being sick, result from wrong doing, outside forces, or events that happened close together in time or location. They define illness by what they can actually see or feel and may develop conflicting theories about their illness.

7-12 years. Elementary-school-aged children still understand best that which they can feel or see. By about age nine or ten, they start to understand some of the unobservable active processes of their bodies, but they tend to believe firmly that it is germs that cause illness. At about age 11 or 12 they start to understand the body's own healing process.

Adolescents. Adolescents are increasingly capable of understanding the complexities of how their body operates. Some teens may take an intellectual view of their illness and try to learn as much as possible about it. They may develop their own personal ideas about illness by combining emotion, fact, fantasy and even, still a measure of self-blame. Adolescents may also assert their independence by refusing or sabotaging treatment.

Family Health Interventions

Research by Hepworth and Doherty (1992) and validated by Yuen, Skibinski and Pardeck (2003) summarizes the following points as to the importance of the family in chronic illness. The authors note:

1. The family plays a critical role in health practices of family members.
2. Illness stresses originating inside and outside the family system influence the physical and emotional health of family members.
3. Family beliefs about health and illness are important to successful treatment outcome.
4. Families go thorough predictable states as they confront and deal with illness has an important impact on family members.

5. The family's adaptation to illness has an important impact on family roles and the family system in general. (pp 4-6)

In order to address these factors several interventions are suggested for family health intervention. However, it must be emphasized that interventions must emphasize the fact that the family should be treated as a unit and focus should not be solely directed on the chronically ill child or adolescent although the developmental sequences of the chronically ill child must be considered.

The **structural model** of family intervention (Minuchin, 1974) places emphasis on family organization for family well being. Hierarchy in families is the principle organizing feature.

The **strategic model** of family intervention best represented by Haley (1973) is viewed in the context of how families resolve their problems in relation to their developmental stages. **Behavioral** approaches to family intervention emphasize the importance of adoptive behavior and its functionality to the ecosystem.

In assessing the impact of chronic illness on the family it is important to differentiate each family's response to the illness. The ABCX family crisis (McCubbin & McCubbin) model is instructive here. Behr and Murphy, et al. (1993) note that " Factor A refers to events that have been an impact on the family system. Factor B refers to the family's resources to meet the challenges of these events. Factor C is the family's perception or definition of the events, which indirectly influences the degree of crisis (Factor X) that might occur in the family. Crisis is defined as change in the family system for which the family's previous patterns of response are not adequate." Factor C has particular relevance for families because it establishes the cognitive domains that are open for families and allows them to reframe their crisis. Several areas of intervention are amenable to challenge. Absolutistic thinking (i.e. use of should and must) in thought processes and metaphors such as "this awful" give little leeway for the family to develop resilience and focus on the objective realities of the situation.

Summary

While there are relatively few cures for a chronic illness, the family health approach to practice offers some hope. By offering a concrete strategy, partnership can be drawn with families to enhance the quality of life for the chronically ill child or adolescent.

References

About.com, (2003) Erickson's Eight Stages of Human Development. Retrieved July 25, 2004, from http://psychology.about.com/library/ weekly/aa091500a.htm

Behr, S.K. and Murphy, P.L. (1993). Research progress and promise: the role of perception in cognitive adaptation to disability. In Turnbull, A.P. et al. *Cognitive coping, families and disability* (pp. 152 – 153). Baltimore, Maryland: Paul Brookes Publishing. pp:152-153

Christian, B.J. (1993). Quality of life and family relationships in families coping with their child's chronic illness. In Dr. Funk, S.G., Tornquist, E.M., Champagne, M.T.,

Wiese, R.A., *Key aspects of caring for the chronically ill (pp. 304-312).* New York, NY. Spring publishing.

Dictionary.com, (2003). Retrieved July 25, 2004, from http://dictionary.reference.com/

Faux, S. (1997) Historical overview of responses of children and their families to chronic illness. In Broome, M.E., Knafi, K., Pridham K., Feetam, S. (1997). *Children and families in health and illness,* pp.179-195. Thousand Oaks, CA: Sage Publications.

Haley, J. (1973) Uncommon therapy. New York: Norton Press.

Margaret Potter, (1998) Chronically ill children: A handout for parents. Bethesda, MD: National Association of School Psychologists.

McCubbin, H.I. and McCubbin, M.A. (1998). Family stress therapy and assessment. The T-double ABCX model of family adjustments and adoption. In H.I. McCubbin & A.J. Thompson (Eds.) Family assessment inventories for research and practice (pp. 3-34). Madison: University of Wisconsin – Madison.

McDaniel, S.H., Hepworth, J.H., Doherty, W.J. (1992). Medical family therapy: A bio-psychosocial approach to families with health problems. New York: Basic Books.

Minuchin, S. (1974). Families and family therapy. Cambridge, MA: Harvard University Press

Yuen, F.K.O, Skibinski, G.J., Pardek, J.T. (2003). Family health social work practice: A knowledge and skills casebook (pp. 4 – 6). New York: Haworth Press.

Chapter 10

Lesbian, Gay, Bisexual and Transgender Family Health Issues

Brenda A. Riemer

Jeanne L. Thomas

Family health is manifested by the development of and continuous interaction among the physical, mental, emotional, social, economic and cultural well being of the family and its members (School of Social Work, Southwest Missouri State University, 1996). Lesbian, gay, bisexual, and transgendered individuals and families (LGBT) have unique family health concerns due to heterosexism, not only within society in general, but also among health–care professionals. This chapter identifies policy issues, unique family health–care concerns, and more general concerns that have unique manifestations among LGBT patients, and possible intervention strategies. The focus of this chapter will be on the multidimensional construct of health as it relates to family health on the individual and societal level.

The World Health Organization (WHO) identifies public policies that are sensitive to health and developmental issues, equitable access to health care, community efforts to optimize health, and steps to control community–specific health problems as parameters shaping health. This chapter provides an overview of health–care concerns unique to, or uniquely problematic for, lesbian, gay, bisexual, and transgendered (LGBT) individuals–including LGBT parents, children, and adolescents. The chapter also includes discussion of possible means of ameliorating these problems.

Many, though not all, unique family health–related concerns of LGBT individuals stem from heterosexism, the assumption that everyone is–and should be–heterosexual. This destructive "ism" exists in our society at large, as well as among family health–care professionals. The issue is compounded for LGBT parents, children, and teenagers. Popular images of "the family" are predominantly heterosexual, and the typical assumption is that LGBT individuals are neither married nor parents. Add to this myopia our culture's reluctance to consider childhood sexuality at all–let alone that which is non–heterosexual–and we have a variety of barriers to ready recognition of the health needs of LGBT individuals and parents.

We begin this chapter with a discussion of public policy, followed by consideration of issues related to health – careaccess. The chapter closes with an overview of possible steps that could prevent, or at least minimize, specific health problems, and efforts that communities could undertake to promote and protect health.

Policy and Access Issues

Public Policy

The LGBT population is an inherently diverse group. That population includes individuals who vary in age, race, ethnicity, income, occupation/profession, and education – to name but a few dimensions (Meyer, 2001). Since health is linked to many of these key demographic indicators, researchers and policy makers concerned with LGBT health–related issues face a formidable challenge. Research and policy development must address the health problems of relatively young, affluent, highly educated "guppies" (gay urban professionals); elderly working class and impoverished individuals; LBGT children and adolescents; and LGBT individuals scattered among and beyond these points on the continua. Arguably, considering family health–related concerns in relation to factors other than sexual orientation (e.g., sex, age, income, etc.) might constitute a more logical approach.

We maintain, however, that though there may be "differences that separate them, LGBT people share remarkably similar experiences related to stigma, discrimination, rejection, and violence across cultures and locales" (Myers, 2001, p. 856). For example, 16 states still have sodomy laws that, in effect, define LGBT individuals as criminals. And recent surveys indicate that most contemporary Americans consider homosexuality morally wrong (Dean, et al, 2000). In addition to stigma, absence of relevant information is a common factor impacting health – care for LGBT individuals (Dean et al., 2000). Two recent Institute of Medicine (IOM) reports (*Report on Lesbian Health; Healthy People 2010 Document for LGBT Health*) demonstrate some progress through their very existence. However, despite the inclusion of lesbians, gays, and bisexuals in *Healthy People 2010*, transgender issues were not included. Furthermore, both reports have multiple gaps in data collected from LGB respondents. There are, of course, no data available about unique health concerns of LGBT children, adolescents, and adults who are not open about their sexual orientation.

Until LGBT health research receives local, state, and federal support comparable to health research for other minority groups, lack of relevant data will remain a common thread across the widely varying health–related concerns of the LGBT population. Perhaps more important on a practical level, public policy and health–care practice informed by research also awaits increased support for research in this area.

Access to Family Health Care

In order for health – care services to be truly accessible, these services must be physically available, economically within reach, and culturally acceptable. The LGBT populations do not, as far as we know, encounter unusual problems related to the physical availability of family health–care services. However, obstacles related to economic access and cultural acceptability are well documented (e.g., Feinberg, 2001; Feinberg, 1997). These barriers effectively prevent "LGBT individuals from receiving the screening and prevention services they need, and cause delays in receiving care for acute conditions" (Dean, et al, 2000, p. 106).

Lesbians, gay men, and bisexuals access health – care less often than do heterosexuals (Dean, et al, 2000; Diamant, Schuster, & Lever, 2000; Mautner Project). The cost of these services, or conversely the unavailability of health insurance, is undoubtedly one reason. Many LGBT individuals work part–time or are self–employed, and thus have minimal health insurance coverage or none at all (e.g., Dean et al., 2000). Furthermore, many insurance companies deny insurance to partners of lesbians or gay men. For LGBT individuals denied insurance coverage who are parents, not only their own health but also their children's access to health – care is compromised.

Wolfe (2000) noted that some gay men choose not to use the health–care benefits that their employer does provide because their employer self–insures. Employers that self–insure have access to employee health – care records and claims, and LGBT employees in states with sodomy laws could realistically fear dismissal if those records state their sexual orientation. Similarly, the military's current "don't ask/don't tell" policy could lead to discharge if an LGBT individual disclosed his or her sexual orientation to a health–care professional.

Transgender people face some unique barriers. Wilcox (2001) described the experience of Robert Eads, a biological female who chose to live as a man. Eads died of ovarian cancer because 20 doctors refused to treat him. Feinberg (2001) gave a similar example from hir[1] own life. S/he was refused care in an emergency room and discharged from a hospital, despite her 104°F temperature, because of being transsexual. When s/he was subsequently hospitalized a few weeks later, the staff "refused to work unless "it" was removed from the (female) floor" (p. 898).

Unfortunately, these accounts are not unique instances. Because transgendered individuals have often encountered scorn and disdain from health–care professionals, many are reluctant to seek care. Although transgendered individuals may or may not be lesbian, gay, or bisexual, they still face many of the same discriminatory attitudes and behaviors that LGB individuals face. And unfortunately even health–care professionals who do not express homophobic

---

[1] Hir is the notation that Feinberg uses. S/he is another transgender pronoun used in this chapter.

attitudes have little or no medical training related to ways in which transgendered status does, and does not, affect health and physiological functioning. Clearly, medical education must incorporate training to prepare physicians, nurses, physician assistants, and other primary care providers to treat transgender patients with sensitivity.

Preventing and Controlling Specific Health Problems[2]

A Note on Terminology–The terminology used in this section is a combination of the terms lesbian, gay, bisexual, transgender (LGBT) and the research–specific terms of "women who have sex with women" (WSW) and "men who have sex with men" (MSM).

Lesbians and Bisexual Women

Lesbians and bisexual women are more likely to smoke cigarettes than are heterosexual women (Aaron, Markovic, Danielson, Honnald, Janosky, and Schmidt, 2001; Dean et al, 2000; Gruskin, Gordon, & Ackerson, 2001). A short report in the *Advocate* (2001) points out tobacco advertising strategies aimed at women (e.g., . . . If you want to be tough and butch, light up a smoke. Want to be femme and sexy? Take a long, slow drag and let the smoke curl around your hair [p. 37]). Since cigarette use is closely linked to the incidence of cancers and respiratory disease, lesbians and bisexual women are at a higher risk for these illnesses. Furthermore, these women's children are at increased risk of illnesses associated with passive smoking. These heightened risks are particularly problematic given that LGBT individuals access health care, including routine screening procedures, less often than do heterosexual people (see above).

Lesbians and bisexual women also use alcohol at higher rates than do heterosexual women (Aaron et al., 2001; Gruskin et al., 2001). These trends are moderated by age, however. For all women, the age range most likely to engage in heavy drinking was 20–34 (23.3% of respondents classified as heavy drinkers– at least 60 drinks per month). This percentage dropped to 7.1% for the 35–49 age

---

[2] Because of length limitations, this chapter cannot provide a comprehensive review of all possible health issues for LGBT individuals. We summarize only selected, particularly pressing and/or well-documented unique health concerns. Additionally, other than alcohol and drug use, psychological disorders will only be discussed briefly at the conclusion of the chapter.

range, and then fell to 0% for the 50 and older age range. Abstinence increased for each age range tested. Furthermore, the major difference in drinking behavior related to sexual orientation occurred in the 20–34 age cohort; lesbians and bisexuals over age 50 did not differ in drinking behavior from their heterosexual counterparts.

The most researched topic in lesbian health is breast cancer. Dean et al. (2000) report that lesbians are at a higher risk for breast cancer than heterosexual women due to "higher rates of risk factors such as obesity, alcohol consumption, nulliparity [no children], and lower rates of breast cancer screening" (p. 111). Recall that LGBT individuals access health – care generally at lower rates than do heterosexuals. More specifically, lesbians receive routine gynecological screening exams at lower rates than do heterosexual women (e.g., Marrazzo et al., 2001). Consequently, lesbians receive less frequent screening for breast cancer as well as other cancers of the reproductive system.

It is particularly disturbing that lesbians in recent research have reported being told by a health–care provider that they did not need a Pap test because they were not sexually active with men (Marrazzo et al., 2001). The "myth" of cervical cancer being transmitted (via HPV) only via intercourse with a male partner is a barrier for WSW to receiving appropriate preventative care. The resulting failures to detect reproductive cancers in early stages are, of course, potentially life–threatening. And, to the extent that self–care health practices are socialized in families, it is troublesome to consider the lessons that these lesbians' children may learn–that health–care providers have little to offer them, or that they merit minimal attention from health–care providers.

Lesbians are not at a higher risk than other women for sexually transmitted diseases (STDs). In fact, many STD's are less common among lesbians than among women who have sex with men. However, STDs such as candidiasis and trichomonas vaginalis can be transmitted between women (for a review, please see Dean et al 1999).

Bisexual and Homosexual Men

Like their lesbian and bisexual women counterparts, gay and bisexual men smoke cigarettes and use alcohol more frequently than do heterosexual men. Interestingly, gay men report alcohol–related problems more often than do heterosexuals, even in studies that fail to detect actual differences in drinking behavior (e.g., McKirnan & Peterson, 1989). Therefore, gay men may believe that they drink more heavily than their heterosexual counterparts, even if no such difference exists. As with lesbians' children, gay men's children are potentially exposed to health risks related to passive smoking and problematic alcohol use at greater rates than the children of heterosexual men.

HIV/AIDS is the most widely researched and discussed LGBT health related topic. Some researchers report that high–risk MSM behaviors (e.g., unprotected anal intercourse) have grown more frequent over the past decade (Catania, Osmond, Stall, Pollack, Paul, Blower, Binson, Canchola, Mills, Fisher, Choi, Proco, Turner, Blair, Henne, Bye, & Coates, 2001; Wolitski, Valdiserri, Dennin, & Levine, 2001). The 1999 Gay Men's Health Crisis (GMHC) survey differed from many prior surveys about risk behavior in asking not only whether participants engaged in anal intercourse, but also about whether they had receptive or insertive relations. Even more important, this survey also included questions about condom usage and knowledge of partners' sexual histories and HIV status.

The GMHC results indicated that over the year preceding the survey 15% of the MSM did not engage in anal intercourse, and 35% engaged in anal intercourse with a condom. However, 39% of the respondents had unprotected anal intercourse–a percentage similar to those obtained in other surveys of MSM sexual behavior (see above). Of those respondents who reported engaging in unprotected anal intercourse, fewer partners were reported (relative to those respondents who did not report this practice). Furthermore, HIV negative men more often reported that they practiced insertive relations, perhaps reflecting the belief that HIV is less often transmitted to the insertive partner.

The GMHC (1999) survey also included questions about HIV testing and HIV status. The men least likely to be tested were the youngest and oldest participants (e.g., those under 25 and over 59 years of age), as well as Asian/Pacific Islander men. A relatively small percentage of respondents reported positive HIV status, or that they did not know their HIV status (both 13%); nearly three–quarters of the respondents (73%) were HIV negative. Black and Latino men were most likely to be HIV positive, while Asian/Pacific Islander men were the least likely to be HIV positive. Unfortunately, this survey did not include questions about respondents' parental status, so it is not possible to consider associations among beliefs, practices, and whether respondents had children.

Drug use was addressed in the GMHC (1999) survey. Recreational drug use during sexual relations is important context, as that practice may increase the likelihood of engaging in unprotected intercourse (Quittner, 2001). Some experts caution against that generalization, however (GMHC, 1999). Nearly half (43%) of the sample reported no drug use during sexual encounters. Of the remaining men who reported using drugs and/or alcohol during sexual relations, only a few (2%) reported always using drugs or alcohol during relations. Caucasians (27%) were most likely to use recreational drugs or alcohol during sexual encounters.

Certain cancers are more frequent among gay and bisexual men than among the general male population. Kaposi's sarcoma, Hodgkin's lymphoma, and Hodgkin's disease appear at a higher rate in gay and bisexual men. These conditions, of course, are associated with HIV/AIDS. Additionally, MSM who practice anal intercourse are at increased risk of contracting anal cancer, and two cancer precursors (HPV and ASIL) appear more frequently among MSM versus heterosexual men (Dean et al, 2000).

Gay men are at high risk for contracting hepatitis A and B, reflecting their relatively high rates of drug use and the risks associated with anal intercourse. Thus, hepatitis vaccinations are recommended for gay and bisexual men (Dean et al, 2000). Currently, however, few gay and bisexual men actually are vaccinated against hepatitis. This contrast between recommendation and practice likely stems from the relative infrequency with which gay and bisexual men access health – care (see above) as compared to heterosexual men.

As compared to WSW and heterosexual men, MSM are at a higher risk for many STD's (e.g., syphilis, rectal gonorrhea, genital warts, herpes, HIV infection, urethritis, pharynigitis, and chlamydia) (Dean et al., 1999). Not surprisingly, the rate of STDs in MSM has increased with the decline in reported condom use among MSM identified in recent surveys (see above). As with the population in general, it is difficult to obtain accurate and precise data regarding frequency of STD infection between MSM and bisexual men due to the stigmas attached to both STDs and homosexuality.

Transgender Individuals

The term transgender describes a diverse collection of people. The transgendered population includes "drag queens" who dress as members of the opposite sex, intersexed persons (who possess both male and female sexual characteristics), and transsexuals (who live as members of the opposite sex, and may have completed sex reassignment treatment and/or surgery). The health needs and risks may be very different for each of these individuals. In this chapter we focus on transsexuals. Unfortunately, relatively little research has addressed the needs of transgender individuals, and they are targets of prejudice among health–care professionals (see above).

HIV occurs more frequently among transsexuals than among the general population (Clements–Nolle, K., Marx, R., Guzman, B.A., & Katz, M., 2001). In a recent survey of over 500 transgender individuals (392 male–to–female [MTF] and 121 female–to–male [FTM]), over a third (35%) of the MTF participants were HIV positive, whereas very few (2%) of the FTM participants were HIV positive (Clements–Nolle et al., 2001). This contrast reflects corresponding differences in demographic and behavioral characteristics. Being HIV positive was associated with having multiple partners (over 200) and with injection drug use, both of which were more common among MTF individuals than among FTM individuals; these researchers suggested that the male–to–female transgender individuals may turn to sex work because they face "severe employment

161

discrimination, and this may account for the high number of sexual partners . . .'
(p. 919).

Only 50% of these participants were receiving medical care. Recall that transgendered individuals face particularly difficult barriers to receiving care in the form of ignorance and discrimination among health-care professionals. Economic factors also likely limit access to health-care for transgendered individuals. If in fact employment discrimination and work in the sex trades are relatively common among transgendered people, then health insurance benefits would be correspondingly infrequent among that population.

In general, transsexuals who have sex reassignment surgery are satisfied with the results of their surgery (Dean et al., 1999), and psychological functioning improves after surgery. However, transsexuals may suffer medical complications of hormonal treatments used in conjunction with or instead of surgery. For example, MTF individuals experience blood clots (venous thromboembolism) much more frequently than the general population (Harry Benjamin International Gender Dysphoria Association, 1998). Other side effects of hormone therapy include weight gain, liver disease, and benign pituitary tumors. FTM individuals are at risk for increased lipid and cholesterol levels, heart disease, liver disease, acne, and male pattern baldness.

Promoting and Protecting Health

Though initial steps to identify health–related concerns among the LGBT population have occurred, translating that information into recommendations for community efforts to promote and protect the health of LGBT people and their children is not a straightforward process. As noted earlier, the LGBT population is diverse. Furthermore, definitions of lesbian, gay, bisexual, and transgendered individuals differ as well. And, sexual identity does not always equate with sexual behavior, since some individuals who have homosexual relations may identify themselves as heterosexual. Finally, the implications of all of these issues must be considered in the context of LGBT parents, LGBT children and teens of heterosexual parents, and families in which both parents and children are LGBT.

Certainly, more reliable data about health–related concerns among the LGBT population is needed in order to promote and protect that group's health. Craft and Mulvey (2001) advocate including LGBT individuals in epidemiological studies. They also call for innovative outreach efforts, increased awareness by health – care providers, and training in cultural diversity to staff members/health – care providers. (See Craft & Mulvey, 2001, Table 1 for a complete list of service imperatives.) For example, the Mautner Project for Lesbians with Cancer has provided training for health – care practitioners to improve the care lesbians receive (Mautner Project).

In addition, health – care professionals need to understand and combat the homophobia and heterosexism within their profession. Though the American Medical Association includes sexual orientation in their civil and human rights policies (Schneider, J.S. & Levin, S., 1999), many gay and lesbian medical students experience homophobia (Kirby, 2001) and–as documented earlier in this chapter – instances of homophobia among medical professionals occur. Feinberg (2001) makes excellent suggestions about transgender health – care that would improve health – care for all LGBT individuals. These suggestions include referring to patients by their full names (rather than by sex–specific titles), providing unisex bathrooms and equipment, providing on–site patient advocates, and supporting community–based research. Similarly, gay men and lesbians in London reported prejudice from health professionals. One suggestion given in the study is to teach doctors in medical school about gays and lesbians as part of diversity training (Lles, 2003).

In short, heterosexism and homophobia need to be dealt with as any other form of prejudice (e.g., racism, anti–Semitism) in health – care settings. The professions themselves need to insure that these forms of prejudice are considered unprofessional, unethical, and unacceptable. Not only by enacting written policy but also by developing professional and institutional cultures and mores, physicians, nurses, and health – care administrators are obligated to develop peer pressure as well as formal policy to insure equitable and respectful behavior towards all patients.

Development of such formal and informal codes of professional conduct will go a long way toward insuring greater access to health – care for LGBT individuals. At least as important, however, are broader policy and legislative steps to remove economic barriers to care. Decriminalization of homosexual relations under state law and military policy, broadening of employee benefit policies to cover homosexual partners, and the like are critically needed to eliminate financial impediments to health – care for LGBT people. Thus, addressing the health–care rights of LGBT individuals is but one facet of the much larger task of addressing the *human* rights of all individuals.

References

Aaron, D.J., Markovic, N., Danielson, M.E., Honnold, J.A., Janosky, J.E., & Schmidt, N.J. (2001). Behavioral risk factors for disease and preventive health practices among lesbians. *American Journal of Public Health, 91*(6), 972–975.

Adams, B. (2001). Lost in the smoke. *The Advocate,* (May 22), 37.

Catania, J.A., Osmond, D., Stall, R.D., Pollack, L., Paul, J.P., Blower, S., Binson, et al. (2001). The continuing HIV epidemic among men who have sex with men. *American Journal of Public Health, 91* (6), 907–914.

Craft, E.M., & Mulvery, K.P. (2001). Addressing lesbian, gay, bisexual, and transgender issues from the inside: One federal agency's approach. *American Journal of Public Health, 91*(6), 889–891.

Dean, L., Meyer, I., Robinson, K., Sell, R.L., Sember, R., Silenzio, V.M.B., et al. (2000). Lesbian, gay, bisexual, and transgender health: Findings and concerns. *Journal of the Gay and Lesbian Medical Association, 4*(3), 101–151.

Diamant, A.L., Schuster, M.A., & Lever, J. (2000). Receipt of preventive health care services by lesbians. *American Journal of Preventive Medicine, 19*(3), 141–148.

Feinberg, L. (2001). Trans health crisis: For us it's life or death. *American Journal of Public Health, 91*(6), 897–900.

Feinberg, L. (1997). *Transgender warriors: Making history from Joan of Arc to*

Dennis Rodman. Boston: Beacon Press.

Gay and Lesbian Medical Association and LGBT health experts (2001). *Healthy people 2010 companion document for lesbian, gay, bisexual, and transgender (LGBT) Health.* San Francisco, CA: Gay and Lesbian Medical Association.

Gay Men's Health Crisis (1999). *Sexual health survey.* New York: GMHC.

Gruskin, E.P., Hart, S., Gordon, N. & Ackerson, L. (2001). Patterns of cigarette smoking and alcohol use among lesbians and bisexual women enrolled in a large health maintenance organization. *American Journal of Public Health, 91*(6), 976–979.

Harry Benjamin International Gender Dysphoria Association (1998). *The Standards of Care for Gender Identity Disorders.* Dusseldorf: Symposion Publishing.

Kirby, D. (2001). The out interns. *The Advocate,* (May 22), 33–34.

Lles, A. (2003). Student BMJ, 11, 355.Lombardi, E. (2001). *Enhancing transgender health care. American Journal of Public Health, 91*(6), 869–872.

Marrazzo, J.M., Koutsky, L.A., Kiviat, N.B., Kuypers, J.M. & Stine, K. (2001). Papanicolaou test screening and prevalence of genital human papillomavirus amog women who have
sex with women. *American Journal of Public Health, 91*(6), 947–952.
Mautner Project. *Removing the barriers to accessing care for lesbians.* Retrieved July 26, 2004, from www.mautnerproject.org/barriers.html.

McKirnan, D.J., & Peterson, P.L. (1989). Alcohol and drug use among homosexual men and women: Epidemiology and population characteristics. *Addictive Behavior, 14,* 545–553.

Meyer, I.H. (2001). Why lesbian, gay, bisexual, and transgender public health? *American Journal of Public Health, 91*(6), 856–858.

Healthy People 2010 (2000). Vol 1 and 2. 2nd ed. Washington, D.C.: US Department of Health and Human Services.

Quittner, J. (2001). All mixed up. *The Advocate,* (May 22) 36.

Schneider, J.S. & Levin, S. (1999). Uneasy partners: The lesbian and gay health
– care community and the AMA. *MSJAMA: The Journal of the American
Medical Association, 282,* 1287–1288.

School of Social Work, Southwest Missouri State University (1996). *A working
paper on family health.* Springfield, MO: Author

Solarz, A.L. (1999). *Lesbian health: Current assessment and directions for the
future.* Washington, D.C.: Institute of Medicine: National Academy
Press.

Wilcox, J. (2001). Editor's note. *American Journal of Public Health, 91*(6), 897.

Wolfe, D. (2000). Men like us: The GMHC complete guide to gay men's sexual,
physical and emotional well–being. New York: Ballantine Books.

Wolitski, R.J., Valdiserri, R.O., Denning, P.H., & Levine, W.C. (2001). Are we
headed for a resurgence of the HIV epidemic among men who have sex
with men? *American Journal of Public Health, 91*(6), 883–888.

Chapter 11

Children of Violence: Family Health in Troubled Families

Joan C. McClennen

The term "domestic violence" has euphemistically been used to describe the abuse of power of adults toward their intimate partners with, usually, females as victims of male perpetrators (Jones, 1994). Increasingly, the term "Intimate Partner Violence" (IPV; CDC, n.d.) is being used in an effort to keep violence against one's intimate partner on the same level as "child abuse" and "elderly abuse." The term "partner" differentiates this type of violence from others, and the term "intimate" is inclusive of any intimate relationship regardless of the couple's marital status or gender.

Initially, research, policies, and programs focused on the female victims and the male perpetrators of IPV. Over that last two decades an increasing amount of attention has been directed toward children witnessing IPV in realization of the highly correlated relationship between the occurrences of IPV and child abuse and of the recognition of the adverse effects on these children's cognitive, emotional, social, and behavioral development resulting from their being witnesses. Children witnessing IPV have been "called the 'silent,' 'forgotten,' and 'unintended' victims. . . " (Edleson, n.d., para. 3). By the turn of the century, literature had sufficient evidence of the incidences and effects on children who witnessed IPV to have this phenomena be considered as a major social problem and to have legislators begin including witnessing of IPV by children as a form of child abuse (Edelson, Mbilinyi, Beeman, & Hagemeister, 2003).

History of Abuse to Women and Children in American Society

Historically, in a patriarchal society, women and children were considered as chattel having little, if any, importance in family decisions. Despite 100 years of being legally free from beatings from their husbands, women remained relatively quiet about the abusive affairs in their homes. In the 1970s, the abuse to women by their intimate partners finally came to the forefront largely due to the feminist movement. Publications revealed the silent terrorism happening to women at the hands of their male partners, the first battered women's shelter was opened, and the National Organization of Women formed the first task force to examine intimate partner violence (IPV).

In relatively synchronized timing, abuse to children at the hands of their caretakers gained societal attention. By 1975, the Children Abuse & Neglect Act created Child Protective Services, and legislative policies and programs were established for the protection of children against violence by their caretakers. The abuse of one family member to another was being un-closeted.

Definition of Children Witnessing Intimate Partner Violence

Typically, "children witnessing IPV" are considered as being those children who are "eyewitnesses" of the abuse; however, children who may not visually observe, but hear, the abuse also need to be included in this definition. Expanding the definition further, children who are used by perpetrators of IPV (e.g., holding them hostage or telling the mothers that their children will be taken if they report the abuse) are "child witnesses" of IPV (Edleson, n.d.). Since emotional abuse is a type of IPV, children witnessing marital discord (e.g., yelling and other forms of non-physical violence) may also be included in this definition. The definition, studies, effects, and any other considerations of children witnessing IPV need to include both eyewitnesses and non-eyewitnesses of physical and non-physical IPV (Edleson, n.d.; Smith, O'Connor, & Berthelsen, 1996).

The Relationship between Intimate Partner Violence and Child Abuse

The overlap between intimate partner violence (IPV) and child abuse has been estimated at 30% to 60% of families (Edleson, n.d.; Smith, et al, 1996). Some of this abuse is caused by the children's attempt to intervene between the adults when the perpetrators' acts of abuse actually were directed at the adult victims (Dobash 1977 as cited in McKay, 1994). In fact, 63% of imprisoned youngsters between the ages of 11 and 20 are guilty of intervening between the adults to the point of killing the perpetrator (NCHDBW, 1994).

Between 35.2% (Smith, et al., 1996) and 70% (Edleson, 1999) of male perpetrators of IPV also abuse their children. As compared with children in families not experiencing IPV, child abuse is 15 times more likely to occur in families experiencing IPV (McKay, 1994). As the severity of the IPV increases, the severity of the abuse to the children increases (Bowker, Arbitell, & McFerron, 1988). Clearly, IPV is a correlate (Gleason, 1995), if not a predictor, of child abuse (McKay, 1994).

Incidence of Child Witnesses

The estimated number of children witnessing IPV has commonly been estimated to be 3.3 million (Straus, 1992 as cited in Edleson, n.d.). Since this estimate was on children under three years of age who were eyewitnesses to physical violence, this estimate is conservative (Edleson, n.d.). In his later study, Straus (1992 as cited in Edleson, n.d.) estimated that 10 million teenagers witness IPV and that one-third of all children witness some form of IPV. Based on one-third of all children, the estimated number of children witnessing IPV translates into approximately 23.7 million (U.S. census, n.d.).

Family Health and IPV

Intimate Partner Violence (IPV) subjugates every part of family health—the physical, mental, emotional, social, economic, cultural, and spiritual dimensions—for each member of the family and the family as a whole (Yuen & Pardeck, 1999). In addition to the bruises resulting from abusive acts, the physical health of all members of the family is jeopardized whether the symptoms are diagnosed or psychosomatic. Mental development of children and victims is hampered by the family havoc. Existing psychological problems and newly developed ones intensify with every abusive act. Abusive families tend to be closed systems, thus depriving the family of healthy social relationships with persons outside of the immediate members. Increased medical expenses, behavioral problems, substance abuse, and employment difficulties are some of the economic costs associated with IPV. Spiritual development is highly unlikely in this atmosphere of fear, anxiety, isolation, and familial cultural chaos. As IPV tends to be intergenerational, without effective intervention, children raised in abusive homes continue the cycle of IPV with all its unhealthy dimensions.

Factors Influencing the Impact of Children Witnessing IPV

The adverse impact on children who witness IPV is reported in empirical studies by numerous authors (Markward, 1997; Smith et al., 1996) and in extensive reviews of the literature (Edleson, n.d.; Wolak & Finkelhor, 1998). When researching, assessing, intervening, or in any other manner considering the cognitive, emotional, social, and behavioral problems resulting from children's witnessing IPV, multiple variables require investigation and control.

Two of these variables are abuse to the children by their caretaker and other types of violence experienced by the children. For children witnessing IPV, the impact can be devastating when compounded by their experiencing violence in their community and viewing violence in the media (Edleson, n.d.). Although some debate exists, children who are both witnesses to IPV and are victims of abuse in their homes exhibit even more serious consequences than do children who have only witnessed IPV (Davis & Carlson, 1987).

The impact on children can be altered depending on family stressors. An increase in behavior problems and a decrease in social competence are reported for children as their mothers' experience increased stress, a higher number of negative life events, and higher frequencies of violence from the perpetrators (Wolfe, Jaffe, Wilson, & Zak, 1985).

170

Evidence exists that the age and gender of children influences the impact of their witnessing IPV (Wolak & Finkelhor, 1998). In general, literature reports girls experience more internalized problems (anxiety and depression) partially due to their increased likelihood of being victims of abuse, and boys experience externalized problems (behavioral) including aggressive acts toward perpetrators of IPV (Dobash, 1977 as reported in Bowker, et al., 1988; Edleson, et al., 2003). Regardless of their age or gender, children witnessing IPV are learning dysfunctional relationship patterns, which will result in intergenerational transmission of violence if intervention is not provided (Hurley & Jaffe, 1990).

The impact on children witnessing IPV is influential in determining their responses to the IPV. In interviewing 114 battered mothers gathering information about their children's intervention responses to IPV (e.g., yelling or becoming physically involved), Edleson, et al. (2003) reported numerous factors determining whether children intervened and the intensity of the intervention. Decreased intervention occurred for children whose mothers were married, well educated, and/or employed and if the children were biologically related to the perpetrator. Intervention increased for children living alone with their mothers. Women in transitional housing, as compared with those in more stable housing, reported a higher rate of intervention by their children. Intervention increased for older children especially, as the intensity of the abuse increased.

In summary, some of the factors determining the impact on children witnessing IPV are the children's age, gender, biological relationship to the perpetrators, and exposure to other forms of violence; the children being victims of abuse; mothers' education, employment, living conditions, martial status, and stress level; and the frequency and intensity of the abuse.

Effects on Children Witnessing IPV

Although children vary considerably in their reactions to witnessing IPV, certain types of problems may be observed depending on their age and gender. While being aware of these stereotypical reactions, professionals need to assess and provide treatment modalities to each child as an individual rather than anticipating certain problems. In a counseling environment, every child needs to be assessed for potential violence in the home (Hurley & Jaffe, 1990).

Infants

Using measures of the heart rate and galvanic skin responses, evidence exists of stress to the fetus due to IPV resulting in severe physiological distress after birth (Sudermann & Jaffe, 1999). Because IPV often occurs when women are pregnant (McFarlane, Parker, Soeken, & Bullock, 1992 as cited in Sudermann and Jaffe, 1999), fetuses are often physically injured, or miscarried. (Sudermann & Jaffe).

According to Erikson's (1963) developmental stages, from birth to three years of age the child is developing basic trust and autonomy. As women struggle with their own physical, emotional, and physiological needs while experiencing IPV, they are hampered in providing the attention and patience to their infants that is so vital during this stage of life. The results may be the infants' failure to thrive, "prolonged crying, irritability, difficulty sleeping, and disruption in eating and play/exploration" (Sudermann & Jaffe, 1999, p. 347).

Preschoolers

Preschoolers are increasingly aware of the IPV within the home and, while continuing with the problems developed during infancy, they may begin manifesting an increase in negative reactions. Often, children of this age behave aggressively including their attempts to intervene during the violent incidences (Edleson, n.d.; Wolak & Finkelhor, 1998). Children may experience problems with enuresis, inappropriate social skills both with adults and peers, somatic complaints, and regression to earlier levels of development (Davis & Carlson, 1987; Wolak & Finkelhor, 1998). At this developmental stage in life they may begin self-blame for the violence in the home (Smith, et al., 1996).

School-age Children

Young children may continue to blame themselves for the IPV and manifest more intense cognitive, emotional, social, and behavioral reactions. They may increase their aggressive behaviors; withdraw with anxiety, depression, and low self-esteem; perform poorly academically; interact inappropriately with their social skills, thus being rejected by their peers; and suffer sleeplessness, eating disorders, and psychosomatic symptoms (Wolak & Finkelhor, 1998). As compared with children not witnessing IPV, those children who do witness are twice as likely to be admitted to the hospital and are twice as often absent from school for health problems (Edleson, et al., 2003). Aggression among siblings is common including biting, spitting, slapping, and numerous other forms of abuse imitative of their observations of IPV and their learning violence as a means to settle conflict (Hurley & Jaffe, 1990). These children grow up confused about the meaning of love, violence, and intimacy (Wolak & Finkelhor, 1998).

Adolescents

Adolescent witnesses of IPV evidence a higher rate of delinquency, assaults, runaways, drug and alcohol abuse, immaturity, personality disorders, and suicide than adolescents who have not witnessed IPV (Davis & Carlson, 1987; Wolak & Finkelhor, 1998). Internalized symptoms may be manifested through depression and low self-esteem (Edleson, n.d). Adolescent boys often resort to aggression as means for problem solving and have a 2,000% greater probability of becoming perpetrators of IPV than non-witnessing boys (NCHDBW, 1994). Throughout their development youth witnesses have shown signs of Posttraumatic Stress Disorder (PSTD). These youth may experience headaches, nightmares, shakiness, feelings of numbness, inability to remember important aspects of events, and exaggerated startle responses (Silvern & Kaersvang, 1989; Wolak & Finkelhor, 1998). As PSTD is not uncommon for children witnessing IPV, professionals need to provide intensive assessment to determine its presence as well as providing appropriate interventions (Lehmann, 2000).

Although some children are more resilient to witnessing IPV than others, in most literature the findings support at least some type of detrimental effect on these children. The responsibility of identifying children experiencing IPV in their homes lies with all professionals and laypersons suspicious of the existence of IPV or of child abuse. Because of their ongoing responsibilities child protective service workers and counselors in domestic violence shelters have additional responsibility in identifying and providing intervention to children witnessing IPV.

Social Workers in Child Abuse and in IPV Systems

On behalf of children witnessing IPV, the Family Health Perspective (Pardeck & Yuen, 1999) requires social workers and other helping professionals to identify and assess all family members for intrapersonal symptoms, interpersonal deficiencies, and environmental stressors. Following a thorough biopsychosocial-spiritual assessment, interventions are required to enhance individuals' well-being as influenced by their family system and social ecology (Yuen & Pardeck, 1999). Early identification of IPV could reduce, if not prevent, adverse effects on child witnesses.

Children's Protective Services has come under criticism for failure to identify and to intervene with child witnesses of IPV (Humphreys, 1999). While investigating cases of reported abuse, workers often avoid or minimize the existence of IPV within the home and thus fail to provide services to child witnesses. This is especially true with families of color (Humphreys, 1999). Concentration is placed on abuse of the child, seemingly discounting the relationship between child abuse and IPV. If abuse is unfounded, all services are discontinued, leaving the family living with the violence in their home.

Children's Protective Service has been responsible for inadvertently encouraging the continuance of IPV through efforts to promote family reunification (Stanley, 1997). When the family is being investigated for child abuse, women lack trust in their social workers and fail to share family problems. In fear of having their children removed, abused mothers maintain the secrecy of IPV, thus, being in "triple jeopardy"—the male perpetrators continue IPV, children remain in the home, and women cope with their own trauma (Stanley, 1997, p. 140).

Failing to use a family-health perspective, Children Protective Services is guilty of not including the male figure in the home in the assessment and intervention processes. The males, whether or not they are perpetrators of violence, are treated as if they were "invisible" (Stanley, 1997, p. 140). Rather

174

than requesting assistance from other workers or law enforcement, social workers have ignored the male in the home in fear of their safety from a potentially violent man (Stanley, 1997).

Women who leave their abusers and seek protection within shelters place themselves and their children in a different, but safe, traumatic situation. These women depend on social workers within the shelters to assist them with the many decisions and actions needed to help them obtain a healthy family lifestyle. Social workers in these shelters have been noted to use inappropriate strategies based on false assumptions. Battered women often are assumed to suffer from learned helplessness, meaning they are unable to protect themselves and their children. Many workers fail to recognize that these women are not passive victims but are trapped by their perpetrators as well as by the system (Dobash & Dobash, 1992 as cited in Stanley, 1997). Empowerment strategies are needed to assist women in the revealing of the IPV and in their taking action appropriate for them and their children.

Even when using empowerment strategies, shelter workers place most energy on helping adult victims. The assessments and interventions needed to help the children are seldom provided. For the adults who return to their homes, services are no longer available to them from social workers knowledgeable about IPV (Stanley, 1997).

In violation of the family health perspective requiring collaboration between social workers and allied professionals, the social service system in place to protect children from abuse in their homes and the system in place to protect victims of IPV are failing to coordinate their efforts toward discontinuing family violence (Humphreys, 1999; Stanley, 1997; Yuen & Pardeck, 1999). Child Protective Services needs to increase their knowledge about IPV, enabling them to identify and to provide intervention for all family members. Likewise, social workers in shelter programs for victims of IPV and social workers in treatment programs for perpetrators need increased sensitivity to the multiple aspects of IPV and its adverse impact on children. Resources are needed for each member of the family and the family as a whole.

Assessment of Child Witnesses

Assessments using the family health approach are based on the biopsychosocial-spiritual functioning of each family member and the family as a whole and are focused on the context within which problems are occurring (Yuen & Pardeck, 1999). Licensed Clinical Social Workers (LCSWs), and other equally trained professionals, conduct accurate and thorough assessments gathering data on all dimensions of each family member's life.

Based on the family-health approach, the principal source of beliefs about health and behaviors is the family as they are the ones making sense of their experiences. During the assessment social workers and the family work in conjunction with one another to assure the family members are active participants and are empowered to define and clarify their presenting problems as well as reflect on those problems identified by the social worker. Professionals must be free of myths and prejudices, knowledgeable about diverse cultures, and aware of the family's present stage of their life course.

A pervasive myth is that IPV occurs only in lower-income homes. In reality, IPV is so insidious that it has no boundaries—economic, spiritual, racial, educational, or any other characteristic known to humankind. In assessing for domestic violence and its danger to child witnesses, professionals need to dispel the myth that IPV does not occur in middle-to-upper socioeconomic families (Owens-Manley, 1999; Weitzman, 2000). All families appearing before counselors can, and should be, assessed for the existence of violence in the home (Hurley & Jaffee, 1990; Limandri & Sheridan, 1995).

The most immediate determinant of the assessment process is to conduct lethality assessments of the adults and to provide protection for victims of IPV and their children. Lethality assessments can determine the extent of danger to the children and the advisability of the children being with one or both adults. Verbal communication, observations, and assessment instruments can assist in determining the existence and the extent of violence in the home as well as predictive risk factors for violence.

One of the most commonly used tools for assessing the existence and extent of family violence is the Conflict Tactics Scale, which has various versions depending upon the age of the participant (Straus, 1979). A myriad of other assessment tools are available for social workers. Fischer and Corcoran (1994), Hudson (1992), and Daley (1999) are excellent sources for hundreds of tools for clinical practice. In addition to assessing directly for violence, tools are available for determining the existence of risk factors associated with IPV such as violence in the perpetrator's family of origin, excessive alcohol or drug use, antisocial traits, and generalized aggression (Saunders, 1995). These tools are readily assessable and easy to use in a clinical setting.

In addition to tools, the existence of IPV can be determined using verbal and non-verbal communication of all family members. Children are often more difficult to assess based on their perceived power as being less than the parents and on their limited verbal abilities. During the assessment, interacting with the children is a vital part of assessing for violence in the home. Children will often demonstrate subtle symptoms such as the need to protect their mother against the perpetrator or, mimicking the perpetrator, the use of abusive verbal behavior toward their mother.

Children can be asked about their attitudes as to means of resolving conflict as well as their actions in dealing with violent incidents; children who have witnessed IPV will resort to socially inappropriate responses in these areas (Saunders, 1995). Children can be asked about, "How and when violence occurs, who gets hurt, how often and how family members protect themselves from anger outbursts" (Hurley & Jaffe, 1990, p. 474). Other questions include what the child does when violence occurs, what s/he will do if it reoccurs, and the location of safe places where violence does not occur.

When assessing for violence within the family, the intrapersonal and interpersonal problems of all children in the home need attention. Observing and talking with siblings is essential. Siblings living in violent homes vacillate between protection of and violence toward one another, and their problem-solving skills are most often the use of violent acts. As these children tend to be jealous of one another, these violent acts are frequent (Hurley & Jaffe, 1990).

Of immense importance in the assessment process is teaching victims and children safety planning (Wolack & Finkelhor, 1998). Included in the safety plans for adult victims are items to have packed and hidden for an escape, telephone numbers to call for help, and a way to escape the perpetrator. Safety plans for children include means of escaping future episodes of violence between the adults by knowing safe places to hide, people they can call for help, and other resources available to them. These steps should be role played by adult victims and children in preparation of future episodes. Prevention of further exposure to experiencing IPV is crucial in minimizing any further harm to family members.

When IPV exists in the home, couples wanting to remain together require assessment for their commitment to the relationship and to stopping the violence (Hurley & Jaffe, 1990). Violence against another person is a criminal offense and must stop immediately. Perpetrators must be willing to attend group treatment specifically designed for perpetrators of IPV. Victims need to learn means to protect themselves and to become empowered to adopt a healthier lifestyle. Couples wanting to remain together must be willing to continue counseling.

Couples are to explore issues of custody and support if they do not want to remain together or if they are deemed inappropriate to remain together. Commitment to stopping the violence remains imminent. Resources are needed for all members of the family—whether or not they continue their relationship.

The assessment requires a multi-method approach (O'Leary & Murphy, 1999). Additional techniques can be used during the assessment such as ecomaps diagramming the family's current connections with the environment and genograms for identifying intra-familial patterns over time (Paquin & Bushorn, 1993). The assessment combines information from all parties—verbal, observations, instruments, and data from any other sources (past records and other individuals).

In the assessment process, social workers must be mindful of their being governed by legal policies and ethical standards. Before beginning the counseling

178

sessions, social workers are wise to have a written agreement with their clients that include their legal responsibility to report suspected child abuse. Despite the negative impact to children, only a few states include being a witness of IPV within their statues addressing child abuse (Susi, 1998).

Assessment Instruments

Despite their ease of acquisition and use, many counselors are resistant to using measuring instruments in their assessments of family functioning (Daley, 1999). These instruments can be helpful in providing guidelines for effective intervention. Recommendations for assessment instruments include

- A Survey of Children's Exposure to Community Violence (Martinez & Richters, 1993 as cited in Wolack & Finkelhor, 1998): an assessment of children's exposure to any type of violence.

- Child Behavior Checklist (Achenback & Edelbrock, 1983 as cited in McClennen, 2003): an assessment of various kinds of symptoms and problem areas.

- Children's Impact of Traumatic Events Scale (Briere, 1996 as cited by McClennen, 2003): an assessment of trauma and its impact.

- Youth Self Report Form (Achenbach, 1991): an assessment of the overall adjustment of the child.

- Trauma Symptom Checklist for Children (Briere, 1996): an assessment for measuring anxiety, depression, anger, under-and overarousal, dissociation, and sexual concerns.

- McMaster Model of Family Functioning (Milller, Epstein, Bishop, & Keitner, 1985 as cited in Daley, 1999): an assessment of family functioning in all settings on such issues as their ability to problem-solve, communicate, and cooperate.

- Family Resilience Model (McCubbin, Thompson, & McCubbin, 1996 as cited in Daley, 1999): as assessment of families' ability to handle stressors and problem solve.

Intervention

The assessment of the family will determine whether intervention is necessary and the type of intervention to pursue. Intervention also depends upon the placement of the children (e.g. whether they are in shelters) and alternative supportive resources for the children (e.g., relatives). Equifinality within the family health approach purports numerous ways exists to reach the same point of discontinuing family violence (Friedrich, 1996). The ultimate goal of intervention is to develop and maintain healthy states for all family members.

Social workers assume numerous roles in helping the family system within the social ecology. As a primary source of assistance to clients, they are the conferees. They are brokers while linking family members to outside sources and advocates when outside sources are resistant to the needs and requests of the family.

Social workers view communities as critical in providing support for the family. Family members need to exchange isolation for interaction with outside sources. Adverse community conditions require social workers' intervention as a social planner and a locality developer.

Micro- and Mezzo-levels of Intervention

No one professional can solve all the problems involved with family violence. In abusive situations each adult member of the family is treated separately. Intermittently couples and families can meet together as a barometer of their present status. Victims can benefit from shelters that provide group counseling for sharing with other individuals experiencing their same problems. Perpetrators need to attend a batterers' program where they can learn about power and control and alternative means of problem solving while sharing with individuals experiencing similar problems of unhealthy family interactions.

Working with children who have witnessed IPV begins with building rapport. Cognitive, physical, and social problems are to be verbally revealed by the children when they are ready. The existence and extent of these problems will develop as the trust increases between the child and the counselor.

Pre-school children witnessing IPV often require social distance to prevent exacerbating their anxiety (Ragg & Webb, 1992). Helpful in having them alleviate the impact of witnessing IPV is the use of human and animal doll families, aggressive human and animal doll figures, human and animal puppets, drawing materials, telephones, and tactile materials. Bibliotherapy is also helpful in teaching them to identify and express feelings, and resolve problems (Tutty & Wagar, 1994).

During the abuse-focused aspect of treatment, children are to be assisted in exploring various aspects of their trauma. The process includes identifying people and places in which the children feel safe, revealing the secrets that the children have promised to keep in relation to the existence of the abuse, and exhibiting the extent of damage to their psychosocial development. This is a difficult and often long-term phase but is essential for children's treatment (Karp & Butler, 1996).

Ongoing strategies for assisting these children require repairing children's sense of self, processing feelings of guilt and shame associated with the trauma, and learning new, appropriate coping skills. The final stages move children into becoming future oriented and empowered over their future. These processes require a counselor who is experienced in working with children; prevention is required to avoid unhealthy transference and countertransference between the counselor and the children (Karp & Butler, 1996).

Group therapy has been found to be effective in alleviating the trauma of having witnessed IPV (Allessi & Hearn, 1998; Hurley & Jaffe, 1990; Ragg & Webb, 1992). For children in shelters, crisis and short-term intervention is most feasible considering the lack of stability within the family. Even six sessions can help children identify feelings, improve problem-solving skills, and learn healthy interpretation of love and intimate relationships. On-going group counseling can assist children in coping with their feelings of fear, sadness, and anger and challenging attitudes about aggression and family behaviors that promote violence (Davis & Carlson, 1987; Hurley & Jaffe, 1990).

Macro-level Intervention

The elimination of problems resulting from children witnessing IPV accompanies the discontinuation of IPV itself and, at best, is formidable. A multidisciplinary, community-wide approach, such as the one recommended by the Coordinated Approach to Reducing Family Violence Conference, is recommended (Witwer & Crawford, 1995). This approach includes identifying, pursuing, and obtaining long-term funding for interventions, having specialists and advocates in all practice settings, and maintaining a comprehensive management information system. This coordinated effort requires commitment not only from the personnel of the criminal justice system, social workers, school personnel, personnel from domestic violence programs, and other professionals commonly associated with family violence, but also the effort requires cooperation of media, business persons, and all community citizens interested in stopping family violence.

Treatment Barriers

Information about effective treatment of children witnessing IPV appears scant in comparison to literature on other issues about IPV. One reason may be that most research of IPV uses as its sample women and their children who are in shelter programs, thus, eliminating information about the women and children not using these programs. Other reasons for lack of information are barriers to receiving treatment experienced by women in shelters. Some of these barriers are identified as technical difficulties (e.g., the women's work schedules conflicting with the times counseling sessions are offered), violence-related stress preventing women from attending treatment sessions, and parents' lack of understanding of the trauma experienced by their children while witnessing family violence (Peled & Edleson, 1999).

Summary

Millions of families are experiencing intimate partner violence (IPV) and the adverse effects to every part of the seven dimensions of well-being—physical, mental, emotional, social, economic, cultural, and spiritual. No persons or families are immune to this criminal act within their own homes. Without effective intervention the effects of IPV can begin before a child is born and continue until death. Systems in place for protecting children and adult victims of family violence lack the resources to maintain a coordinated effort toward returning families to healthy, wholesome, safe sanctuaries. Reducing IPV and the problems experienced by the family members, including the children who witness this violence, requires the committed effort of every professional and layperson.

Recommendations for furthering the efforts toward achieving the goal of stopping IPV are

- form community-wide taskforces for a coordinated effort toward education, prevention, and intervention of IPV;

- coordinate the services of social workers in Children's Protective Services and in IPV shelters;

- take a family health approach when working with families experiencing IPV including providing a thorough biopsychosocial-spiritual assessment of all family members, intervening in the context of the family system, empowering the family to participate in the assessment and treatment processes, following the strengths approach while recognizing stressors caused by various family life courses, cultural diversity, and needed changes in the environment that are detrimental to the families' development;

- conduct research and program evaluations to determine the incidence rates of children exposed to IPV, the effects on these children, and effective intervention approaches to help them and their families;

- implement programs and policies based on the results of this research; and

- include children's witnessing of IPV in the definition of and statutes for the protection of children.

References

Achenbach, T. M. (1991). *Youth self report.* Burlington, VT: University Associates in Psychiatry.

Alessi, J. J., & Hearn, K. (1998). Group treatment of children in shelters for battered women. In A. R. Roberts (Ed.), *Battered women and their families* (2nd ed.) (pp. 159-173). NY: Springer Publishing.

Bowker, L. H., Arbitell, M., & McFerron, J. R. (1988). On the relationship between wife beating and child abuse. In K. Yllo & M. Bograd (Eds.), *Feminist Perspectives on Wife Abuse* (pp. 158-174). Newbury Park, CT: Sage Publications.

Briere, J. (1996). *Trauma symptom checklist for children.* San Antonio, TX: The Psychological Corporation/Harcourt Brace.

Centers for Disease Control and Prevention [CDC]. (nd). Intimate partner violence fact sheet. Retrieved September 27, 2002 from www.cdc.gov/ncipc/factsheets/ipvfacts.htm.

Daley, J. G. (1999). Clinical instruments for assessing family health. In J. T. Pardeck & F. K. O. Yuen (Eds.), *Family Health : A holistic approach to social work practce* (pp. 81–100). Westport, CT : Auburn House.

Davis, L. V., & Carlson, B. E. (1987, September). Observation of spouse abuse: What happens to the children? *Journal of Interpersonal Violence, 2*(3), 278-291.

Edleson, J. L. (1999). The overlap between child maltreatment and woman abuse: Conjugal violence. *Violence Against Women, 5*(2), 134-145.

Edleson, J. L. (n.d.) Children's witnessing of adult domestic violence. Retrieved June 25, 1998 from www. mincava,umn.edu/papers/witness.htm.

Edleson, J. L., Mbilinyi, L. F., Beeman, S. K., & Hagemeister, A. K. (2003). How children are involved in adult domestic violence: Results from a four-city telephone survey. *Journal of Interpersonal Violence, 18*(1), 18-32.

Erikson, E. H. (1963). *Childhood and society* (2nd ed.). New York: Norton.

Fischer, J., & Corcoran, K. (1994*). Measures for clinical practice: A source*

184

book. New York: Free Press.

Friedrich, W. N. (1996). Foreward. In C. L. Karp and T. L. Butler. *Treatment strategies for abused children: From victim to survivor* (pp. xiii-xvi). Thousand Oaks, CA: Sage.

Gleason, W. J. (1995). Children of battered women: Developmental delays and behavioral dysfunction. *Violence and Victims, 10*(2), 153-160.

Hudson, W. W. (1992*). WALMYR assessment scales scoring manual.* Tempe, AZ: WALMYR.

Humphreys, C. (1999). Avoidance and confrontation: Social work practice in relation to domestic violence and child abuse. *Child and Family Social Work, 4,* 77-87.

Hurley, D. J., & Jaffe, P. (1990, August). Children's observations of violence: II. clinical implications for children's mental health professionals. *Canadian. Journal of Psychiatry, 35*(6). 471-476.

Jones, A. (1994). *Next time, she'll be dead: Battering & how to stop it.* Boston, MA: Beacon Press.

Karp. C. L., & Butler, T. L. (1996). Introduction and theory. In C. L. Karp & T. L. Butler (Eds), *Treatment strategies for abused children: From victim to survivor* (pp. xvii-xxvi). Thousand Oaks, CA: Sage.

Lehmann, P. (2000). Posttraumatic stress disorder (PTSD) and child witnesses to mother-assault: A summary and review. *Children and Youth Services Review, 22*(3/4), 275-304.

Limandri, B. J., & Sheridan, D. J. (1995). Prediction of intentional interpersonal violence: An introduction. In J. C. Campbell (Ed.), *Assessing dangerousness: Violence by sexual offenders, batterers, and child abusers* (pp. 1-19). Thousand Oaks, CA: Sage.

Markward, M. J. (1997). The impact of domestic violence on children. *Families in Society: The Journal of Contemporary Human Services*, 66-70.

McClennen, J.C. (2003). Intervening with domestic violence: Using the family
    health perspective. In F. K. O. Yuen, G. J. Skibinski, & J. T. Pardeck
(Eds.), *Family health social work practice: A knowledge and skills casebook* (pp.
65-80), Binghamton, NY: Haworth Press.

McKay, M. M. (1994). The link between domestic violence and child abuse:
    Assessment and treatment considerations. *Child Welfare League of
    America._LXXIII* (1).29-39.

National Clearinghouse for the Defense of Battered Women [NCHDBW]. (1994,
    February*). Statistics pac*ket (3rd ed.). Philadelphia: Author.

O'Leary, K. D., & Murphy, C. (1999). Clinical issues in the assessment of
    partner violence. In R. T. Ammerman & M. Hersen (Eds.), *Assessment of
    family violence: A clinical and legal sourcebook*, (2nd ed.) (pp. 24-47).
    NY:John Wiley and Sons.

Owens-Manley, J. (1999). Battered women and their children: A public policy
    response. *Affilia: Journal of Women & Social Work, 14*(4), [Electronic
    Version] Retrieved October 10, 2001 from
    http://ehostvgw3.epnet.com/fulltext.asp?resultSetId.

Paquin, G. W., & Bushorn, R. J. (1993). Family treatment assessment for
novices. In
    J. B. Rauch (Ed.), *Assessment: A sourcebook for social work practice*
    (pp. 47-58). Milwaukee, WI: Families International.

Pardeck, J. T., & Yuen, F. K. O. (Eds.). (1999). *Family Health: A holistic
    approach to social work practice*. Westport, CT : Auburn House.

Peled, E., & Edleson, J. L. (1999). Barriers to children's domestic violence
    counseling: A qualitative study. *Families in Society: The Journal of
    Contemporary Human Services, 80*(6), (578–586).

Ragg, D. M., & Webb, C. (1992). Group treatment for the preschool child
    witness of spouse abuse. *Journal of Child and Youth Care, 7*(1), 1-19.

Saunders, D. G. (1995). Prediction of wife assault. In J. C. Campbell (Ed.),
    *Assessing dangerousness: Violence by sexual offenders, batterers, and
    child abusers* (pp. 68-95). Thousand Oaks, CA: Sage.

Silvern, L., & Kaersvang, L. (1989). The traumatized children of violent marriages. *Child Welfare League of America, LXVII*(4), 421-436.

Smith, J., O'Connor, I., & Berthelsen, D. (1996). The effects if witnessing domestic violence on young children's psycho-social adjustment. *Australian Social Work, 49*(4), 3-10.

Stanley, N. (1997). Domestic violence and child abuse: Developing social work practice. *Child and Family Social Work, 2*, 135-145.

Straus, M. A. (1979). Measuring family conflict and violence: The Conflict Tactics Scale. *Journal of Marriage and the Family, 41*, 75-88.

Sudermann, M., & Jaffe, P. G. (1999). Child witnesses of domestic violence. In R. T. Ammerman and M. Hersen (Eds.), *Assessment of family violence: A clinical and legal sourcebook* (2nd ed.) (pp. 343-366). NY: John Wiley and Sons.

Susi, P. K. (1998, September/October). The forgotten victims of domestic violence. *Journal of the Missouri Bar, 54*(5), 231-235.

Tutty, L. M., & Wagar, J. (1994). The evolution of a group for young children who have witnessed family violence. *Social Work with Groups, 17*(1/2), 89-104.

U. S. Census Bureau. (n.d.). DP-1. Profile of general demographic characteristics: 2000. Retrieved July 31, 2003 from http://wwwfactfinder.census.gov/servlet/QTTable?ds_name.

Weitzman, S. (2000). *Not to people like us.* NY: Basic Books.

Witwer, M. B., & Crawford, C. A. (1995, October). *A coordinated approach to reducing family violence: Conference highlights.* Washington, DC: U.S., Department of Justice.

Wolfe, D. A., Jaffe, P., Wilson, S. K., & Zak, L. (1985). Children of battered women: The relation of child behavior to family violence and maternal stress. *Journal of Consulting and Clinical Psychology, 53*(5), 657-665.

Wolak, J., & Finkelhor, D. (1998). Children exposed to partner violence. In J. L. Jasinski & L. M. Williams (Eds.), *Partner violence: A comprehensive review of 20 years of research* (pp. 73-112). Thousand Oaks, CA: Sage Publications.

Chapter 12

Healthy Solutions for Immigrant Hispanic Youth
from a Family-Health Perspective

Susan Dollar

Introduction

Hispanics, many of whom are new immigrants, now comprise the largest minority group under the age of eighteen and make up 16% of the youth population in the United States (U.S. Census Bureau, 2000). These youth face many common challenges, including higher rates of poverty, less formal education, and poorer health than their non-Hispanic U.S. counterparts (Anderson-Reardon, Capps & Fix, 2002; Harris, 1999; Dever, 1991; Wilk, 1986). Immigrant Hispanic youth also face the strains associated with resettlement in a new country while dealing with the pressures of adolescent development.

Western models for health promotion often disregard family-health issues, instead focusing on individuals and definitions of health that exclude the family system (Loveland-Cherry, 1996). The family-health social work approach proposed by Pardeck and Yuen (1999) acknowledges the importance of family relationships and behavior in shaping the health of family members. This holistic approach is grounded in an ecological framework which recognizes there are many levels of information that influence health and illness, ranging from an individual's biological makeup, to family influences, to social and environmental factors. Thus, the interaction of family with other systems on multiple levels must be clearly understood for a thorough assessment and effective intervention to take place.

This chapter discusses the effects of immigration on the health of Hispanic youth in relation to the family system. For purposes of this discussion, "family" comprises both immediate and extended family members. In the context of health, the traditional Hispanic family maintains the family unit as a major support system and older family members are consulted for most life decisions, including medical advice, even when formal services are available. Consequently, the family can serve as either a strength or weakness concerning health and wellness, depending upon their level of understanding and willingness to participate in health promotion and fitness. The discussion will adopt a family-health perspective when addressing the best practice methods for improving the health of youth and their families.

Adjustments for Hispanic Youth

Language and cultural factors have a tremendous effect on the ability of the family to adapt to a new environment. Many new immigrants do not speak English as their first language or speak it with limited proficiency (Department of Labor, 1991; Trotter 1988). Cultural factors, such as traditional views of family roles and maintaining their native ethnic identity, also play a role in how families will adopt new values or lifestyles (McGoldrick, 1993). Traditional familial customs and values are often at odds with a Hispanic youth's desire to model the dominant culture's behaviors, attitudes, and values (Waters, 1996; Baptiste, 1993). Given the traditional value placed on family togetherness and respect within the Hispanic culture (McGoldrick, 1993), elders often resist non-kin involvement in family matters (Baptiste, 1993). Intergenerational conflict is normal with the youth's desire to separate and individuate from the family of origin, but many Hispanic families perceive this process as a lessening of parental authority and a rejection of the family and its values (James, 1997; Baptiste, 1993). Rumbaut's study (as cited in James, 1997) reports that immigrant youth struggle with changing ethnic identification. While most choose to self-identify with their parents, some identify as "American" or as a "hyphenated-American"

190

(i.e. Mexican-American). Rumbaut also reports that females tend to choose hyphenated identities more than male youth. With these influences, Hispanic youth face significant stress in adapting to a new world while also dealing with their normal adolescent development (James, 1997).

Overview of Health Risks

Hispanic youth have severely poorer physical health status and less access to health services than non-Hispanic white youth have (Harris, 1999; Dever, 1991; Wilk, 1986). Health disparities and access issues between whites and racial and ethnic minorities are even more pronounced in rural versus urban areas (Sliflkin, R., Goldsmith, L. & Ricketts, T., 2000). Many of the health risks found among Hispanic youth are preventable with early screening, diagnosis, and treatment. National health data suggest a large differential between Hispanics and whites in infectious diseases rates (Anderson-Reardon et al., 2002). Many immigrant youth have undiagnosed illnesses, such as tuberculosis, parasites, and human immunodeficiency virus infection (HIV), congenital syphilis, and hepatitis A and hepatitis B (American Academy of Pediatrics, 1997). There are wide health disparities between whites and Hispanics in the areas of obesity (Kaiser Family Foundation (KFF 2001a) low-birth weight infants (KFF, 2001b), child and adult immunization rates (KFF, 2001c), and asthma, which is the most common severe chronic condition found among Hispanic children (Hernandez, D. & Charney, E., 1998). Diabetes is twice as common among Hispanics as among whites (Kemp, 2003). Dental caries in primary teeth are nearly twice as common among immigrant youth as among their U.S. counterparts (Pollick, Rice & Echenberg, 1987). In addition, many immigrant children are nutritionally deficient and do not meet the current height-for-age and weight-for-age measures when compared with their U.S. counterparts. (Miller, Kiernan, Mathers, Kleinn-Gitelmann, 1995).

The preventable chronic diseases reported among Hispanic adults are a gauge for future health risks among their youth. Major chronic diseases among Hispanic adults include heart disease, cancer, injuries, stroke, homicide, liver disease, pneumonia/influenza, diabetes, HIV infection, and perinatal conditions

(Spector, 1997). Since immigrants' health declines more rapidly as they age than does the health of U.S.-born children, health-prevention efforts should be prioritized to avoid long-term health problems (Anderson-Reardon et al., 2002).

Hispanic youth may also be affected more by psychosocial risks than their U.S. counterparts due to the effects of isolation, poverty and stress, and the lack of mental health care (Kataoka, S., Stein, B., Jaycox, L., Wong, M., Escudero, P., Tu, W., Zaragoza, C., & Fink, A., 2003; National Alliance for Hispanic Health, 2001). Epidemiological data find that depression, low self-esteem, aggression, substance abuse, and academic problems are common among Hispanic youth (Canino, I, Early, B., & Rogler, L., 1980).

Barriers to Receiving Care

Poorer health conditions among Hispanics are exacerbated by their underutilization of health services and mental-health care (McCabe, Yeh, Hough, Landsverk, Hurlburt, Culver, Wells, & Reynolds, 1999; Vega, Kolody, Aguilar-Gaxiola, Catalano, 1999; Bui & Takeuchi, 1992; Angel, 1985). There are a variety of reasons for not seeking health care, including financial (lack of insurance coverage or the financial resources for care), structural (lack of service providers or facilities), and personal (cultural, spiritual, language, lack of knowledge barriers, and concerns about discrimination) (U.S. Department of Health and Human Services, 2000).

Financial Constraints and Lack of Insurance Coverage

Hispanics have the highest uninsured rates of any racial/ethnic group and account for 32.4% of the 43.6 million uninsured Americans reported in 2002 (US. Census Bureau, 2002). This is a critical point since uninsured, low-income families, regardless of race, spend a larger share of income out-of-pocket for health-care services (7 to 11 percent of their income, compared with upper-income families' average of 1 to 2 percent) (Blanton & Correa 1995). In their report, *Racial and Ethnic Disparities in Access to Health Insurance and Health Care,* Brown and other researchers point out that the lack of employer-based coverage accounts for the large differential between whites and Hispanics insured rates, with 43% of Hispanics compared with 73% of whites (Brown, E., Ojeda, V., Wyn R., and Levan, R., 2000).

While the lack of insurance coverage contributes to widening health disparities, Hispanics, regardless of insurance status, are the least likely among all ethnic groups to have a designated provider for health care (Brown et al., 2000). Research shows that racial and ethnic minorities in general are less likely to get regular medical checkups. This fact is troubling when examining the high rates of adult chronic disease that might have been prevented through early screening, diagnosis and management (National Center for Cultural Competence, 2001).

Language and Cultural Barriers

Traditionally, Hispanics prefer natural support systems for medical and other advice, including the extended family, folk healers, religious institutions and merchants' and social clubs (Flaskerud & Calvillo 1991; Scholze, 1990). The primacy of the family unit as a major support system is a strength for many Hispanic families, many of whom are isolated by language barriers and geography (Flaskerud & Calvillo, 1991; Scholze, 1990). Western health service providers are often consulted last when the patient's medical conditions worsen, making diagnosis and treatment more difficult (Spector 1997; Higginbotham, Trevino, & Ray 1990; Reinert 1986). Delays in seeking assistance may also be due to Hispanic families' inflexible work schedules, fear of deportation, difficulty in communication and time orientation, lack of childcare, and inadequate transportation (Lane, 2003; Ramirez & McAlister 1995).

Improving Access to Services from a Family-Centered Perspective

Pardeck and Yuen describe the family-health approach as one that "attempts to help families define, develop, and maintain health states and change non-supportive social environments through micro and macro level interventions" (Pardeck & Yuen, 1999, p. 6). The holistic nature of the family-health approach mirrors common themes within the Hispanic cultures that emphasize client self-determination, the importance of family attachment, the influence of linguistic and cultural differences on access to programs, and the indigenous community's capacity to address their problems through empowerment strategies, such as self-help, outreach education and prevention strategies.

The family's "construction" of health, including definitions of physical, mental, and social well-being, should be defined by each family member to assess their differing beliefs regarding health and wellness. For example, in traditional Hispanic culture, mental stress is not considered an illness that requires seeking assistance outside of the family unit in the same way as acute health problems (Kataoka, S., Stein, B., Jaycox, L., Wong, M., Escudero, P., Tu, W., Zaragoza, C., & Fink, A., 2003). The family system should be tapped as a resource for providing education and support as an important alternative to traditional mental health services. For many Hispanic families, the extended family and a close-knit network of family friends are strong influences on Hispanic youth attitudes toward health promotion and lifestyle. The duty to family, referred to as *carino,* will serve to encourage many family members to involve themselves in healthy education and modeling behaviors (Wood & Price, 1997).

One approach to involving the entire family in health promotion activities is through multicultural family education. Specific topics that can be taught, discussed, and role-played within families include communication and self-esteem skills, and skills to avoid risky behaviors, such as substance abuse, early sexuality, and violence and gang involvement. Multicultural education, which teaches both native and Western practices, should emphasize the impact of disease on the family and the importance of family in promoting healthy behaviors, including health eating and nutrition, exercise, and socializing with family and friends (Wood & Price, 1997).

Agency-based Activities to Reaching Youth and Their Families

Primary prevention and community outreach have been successful means for reaching ethnic minorities and low-income populations. (Atkinson, Thompson, & Grant, 1993). These services should be made available from multiple sources, including schools, churches, health-care providers, housing developments and community-based organizations (Holcomb, Tumlin, Koralek, Capps & Zuberi, 2003). These services should be "user friendly" by providing interpreter services, language phone banks, and translated written materials for those with limited reading proficiency (Holcomb et al., 2003; Smith & Weinman, 1995). Techniques for those with low reading levels, such as story-telling, role-playing, games, and the use of pictures to illustrate ideas can be used to improve comprehension (Werner & Bower, 1984).

Making other adjustments in the service system, to include efforts to recruit and retain bilingual/bicultural staff and to provide ongoing training in Spanish language skills and cultural competency will create a more informed and effective workforce. Actively engaging youth counselors to teach disease prevention and health promotion to their peers is another practical recommendation (Esquivel and Keitel, 1990). In addition, scholarships and other incentives for Hispanic youth to move into health-care, legal and social service professions as future leaders should be provided at the high-school and college levels.

Conclusion

In this chapter, acculturation stress and barriers to health and social services support systems have been discussed as factors that can negatively impact the health and well-being of Hispanic youth and their families. Resettlement to a new country brings significant stress to Hispanic family members. Members differ in their ability to cope with this stress depending upon their personal, linguistic and occupational skills, as well as their financial resources. Intergenerational differences between family members concerning values and beliefs may also compound family stress, leaving youth with the difficult tasks of "fitting in" to a new society while balancing their family's traditional role expectations.

The family-health perspective calls for examining the needs of Hispanic youth within the context of their family circumstances, such as the family's history, structure, roles, strengths and expectations. The importance ascribed to the family by immigrant Hispanics makes it a key change agent in adapting to new social environments and in maintaining health between its members. Involving each family member in the process of health education and disease prevention is an important element to maintaining the family's viability as a central change agent. Service providers can also support Hispanic youth and their families by striving to overcome the cultural, financial and linguistic barriers which exist in the human services and which perpetuate health disparities between Hispanics and the general population.

References

American Academy of Pediatrics (1997). Health care for children of immigrant families, *Pediatrics, 100,* 153-156.

Anderson-Reardon, J., Capps, R. & Fix, M. (2002). The health and well-being of children in immigrant families. *New Federalism: National survey of America's families.* The Urban Institute, newsletter series B, (B-52), 1-7.

Angel, R. (1985). The health of the Mexican-American population. In R.O de la Garza, F.D. Bean, C.M. Bonjean, r. Romo, and r. Alvarez, (Eds.), *The Mexican American experience: An interdisciplinary anthology* (pp. 410-426). Austin, TX: The University of Texas Press.

Atkinson, D., Thompson, C., & Grant, S. (1993). A three-dimensional model for counseling racial/ethnic minorities. *The Counseling Psychologist, 21,* 257-277.

Baptiste, D. A. (1993). Immigrant families, adolescents and acculturation: Insights for therapists. *Marriage and Family Review, 19,* 341-363.

Blanton, L. and A. Correa. (1995). *In the nation's interest: Equity in access to health care: Project on the health care needs of Hispanics and African Americans.* Washington, DC: Joint Center for Political and Economic Studies.

Brindis, C. (1992). Adolescent pregnancy prevention for Hispanic youth: The role of schools, families, and communities. *Journal of School Health, 62,* 345-51.

Brown, E., Ojeda, V., Wyn, R. and Levan, R (2000). *Racial and ethnic disparities in access to health insurance and health care. Los Angeles, CA:* UCLA Center for Health Policy Research. Retrieved September 27, 2003, from http://www.kff.og/content.

Bui, K. & Takeuchi, D. (1992). Ethnic minority adolescents and the use of community mental health care services. *American Journal of Community Psychology, 20,* 403-417.

Canino, I, Early, B., & Rogler, L. (1980). *The Puerto Rican child in New York City: Stress and mental health.* New York, NY: Hispanic Research Center.

Dever, G.E. Alan (1991). Migrant health status: Profile of a population with complex health problems. *Migrant Health Newsline, 8,* 1-16.

Esquivel, G. & Keitel, M. (1990). Counseling immigrant children in schools. *Elementary School Guidance Counseling, 24,* 213-221.

Flaskerud, J.H. and E.R. Calvillo (1991). Beliefs about AIDS, health, and illness among low-income Latina women. *Research in Nursing and Health, 14,* 431-438.

Harris, K. (1999). The health status and risk behaviors of adolescents and immigrant families. In Hernandez, D. (Ed.), *Children of immigrants: Health, adjustment and public assistance* (pp. 286-347). Washington, DC: The National Academies Press.

Hernandez, D. & Charney, E. (1998). *From generation to generation: The health and well-being of children in immigrant families.* Washington, DC: The National Academies Press.

Higginbotham, J.C., E.M. Trevino, and L.A. Ray. (1990). Utilization of curandero by Mexican-Americans: Prevalence and predictors. *American Journal of Public Health, 80,* 32-35.

Holcomb, P., Tumlin, K., Koralek, R, Capps, R., Zuberi, A. (2003). *The application process for TANF, Food Stamps, Medicaid and SCHIP: Issues for agencies and applicants, including immigrants and limited English speakers.* Washington DC, The Urban Institute.

James, D. (1997). Coping with a new society: The unique psychosocial problems of immigrant youth. *Journal of School Health, 67,* 98-103.

Kaiser Family Foundation (2001a). *State health facts online, overweight and obesity rate by race/ethnicity, 2001.* Retrieved September 25, 2003, from http://www..kff.org/cgi-bin/healthfacts

Kaiser Family Foundation (2001b). *State health facts online, rate of low birth weight infants.* Retrieved September 25, 2003, from http://www.statehealthfacts.kff.org/cgi-bin/healthfacts

Kaiser Family Foundation (2001c). *State health facts online, percent of children ages 19-35 months who are immunized by race/ethnicity, 2001.* Retrieved September 25, 2003, from http://www.kff.org/cgibin/healthfacts

Kataoka, S., Stein, B., Jaycox, L., Wong, M., Escudero, P., Tu, W., et al. (2003). A school-based mental health program for traumatized Hispanic immigrant children. *Journal of the American Academy of Child and Adolescent Psychiatry, 42,* 311-318.

Kemp, C. (2003). Mexican & Mexican-Americans: Health beliefs and practices. Retrieved January 6, 2004, from http://www3.baylor.edu/Charles_Kemp/hispanic_health.htm

Lane L. (2003). Meeting the needs of our Hispanic neighbors. *Rural Roads,* 2-7.

Loveland-Cherry, C.J. (1996). Family health promotion and health protection. In P.J. Bomar (Ed.), *Nurses and family health promotion: Concepts, assessment, and interventions* (2nd ed.) (pp. 22-35). Philadelphia, PA: W.B. Saunders Company.

McCabe, K., Yeh, M., Hough, R., Landsverk, J., Hurlburt, M., Culver, S. et al. (1999). Racial/ethnic representation across five public sectors of care for youth. *Journal of Emotional & Behavioral Disorders, 7,* 72-82.

McGoldrick, M. (1993). Ethnicity, cultural diversity, and normality. In Froma Walsh (Ed.), *Normal family processes* (pp. 331-360). New York: The Guilford Press.

Miller, L., Kiernan, M., Mathers, M., & Kleinn-Gitelmann, M. (1995). Developmental and nutritional status of internationally adopted children. *Archives of Pediatric and Adolescent Medicine, 149,* 40-44.

National Alliance for Hispanic Health (2001). *A primer for cultural proficiency: Towards quality health services for Hispanics.* Washington, DC: Author.

National Center for Cultural Competence (2001). *Rationale for cultural competence in primary health care, policy brief 1.* Washington, DC: Georgetown University Center for Child and Human Development. Retrieved September 29, 2003, from http://www.georgetown.edu/research

Pardeck, J.T. & Yuen, F. (1999). *Family Health: A holistic approach to social work practice.* Westport, CT: Auburn House.

Pollick, H., Rice, A., & Echenberg, D. (1987). Dental health of recent immigrant children in the newcomer schools, San Francisco. *American Journal of Public Health, 77,* 731-732.

Ramirez, A.G. and A. McAlister. (1995). Targeting Hispanic populations: Future research and prevention strategies. *Environmental Health Perspective Supplements, 103,* 287.

Reinert, B.R. (1986). The health care beliefs and values of Mexican Americans. *Home Health Care Nurse, 4,* 23-31.

Scholze, J. (1990). Cultural expressions affecting patient care. *Dimensions in Oncology Nursing, 4,* 16-26.

Sliflkin, R.; Goldsmith, L. & Ricketts, T. (2000). *Race and place: Urban-rural differences in health for racial and ethnic minorities.* Working Paper Series No. 66, North Carolina Rural Health Research Program, Cecil G. Sheps Center for Health Services Research. Chapel Hill, NC: The University of North Carolina.

Smith, P. & Weinman, M. (1995). Cultural implications for public health policy for pregnant Hispanic adolescents. *Health Values: The Journal of Health Behavior, Education and Promotion, 19,* 3-10.

Spector, R.E. (1997). *Cultural diversity in health and illness,* (4th ed). Stamford, CT: Appleton & Lange.

Trotter, R.T. (1988). *Orientation to multicultural health care in migrant health programs.* Austin, TX: National Migrant Resource Program.

U.S. Census Bureau (2002). Health Insurance Coverage: 2002. Retrieved May 25, 2004, from http://www.census.gov/prod/2001pubs/p60-215.pdf

U.S. Census Bureau (2000). Current population survey: Population by sex, age,

Hispanic origin, and race.   Retrieved December 29, 2003, from
http://www.census.gov/population/socdemo/hispanic/p 20-535

U.S. Department of Health and Human Services (2000). With understanding
and improving health and objectives for improving health. *Healthy People
2010,* (2nd ed). Washington, DC: US Government Printing Office.

Valdez, R., A. Giachello, Rodriguez-Trias, H, Gomez, P. and de la Rocha, C.
(1993). Improving access to health care in Hispanic communities. *Public
Health Report, 108*, 534-539.

Vega, W., Kolody, B., Aguilar-Gaxiola, S., & Catalano, R. (1999). Gaps in
service utilization by Mexican-Americans with mental health problems.
American Journal of Psychiatry, 156, 928-934.

Waters, M. (1996). Ethnic and racial identities of second generation Black
immigrants in New York City. *International Migration Review, 28,*
749-794.

Werner, D. & Bower, B. (1984). *Helping health workers learn.* Palo Alto, CA:
The Hesperian Foundation.

Wilk, V.A. (1986). *The occupational health of migrant and seasonal
farmworkers in the United States, (* 2nd ed.).   Washington, DC:
Farmworker Justice Fund.

Wood, M. & Price, P. (1997). Machismo and marianismo: Implications for
HIV/AIDS risk reduction and education. *American Journal of Health
Studies, 13,* 44-53.

Chapter 13
Family-Health-Practice Strategies and Techniques to Empower Children and Families in Foster-Care Services

Michele Day

Catherine Hawkins

Mary Ann Jennings

The family-health perspective, which emphasizes the ability of children, adolescents, and families to grow, learn and develop, provides practice principles and strategies that can enhance child-welfare services, including foster-care activities. In family-health practice, the family is the primary context for helping children and adolescents, and it is the family's subjective world view that drives the professional's interventions (Pardeck, Yuen, Daley & Hawkins, 1998). This chapter will explore the relevance of family-health practice principles and strategies for effective substitute care services to children and adolescents and their families.

Family-Health and Foster-care

In the family-health perspective families are the most important sources of stress and comfort for children and youth through various normative developmental transitions (Pardeck & Yuen, 1997). However, a child's removal from his/her family of origin and her/his subsequent placement in foster-care are nonnormative events that impact hundreds of thousands of children each year in the United States. While the biological family often remains a significant source of stress and comfort for children in foster-care, other family forms impact children in substitute care. These family types include nonrelative foster families, kinship/relative families, and adoptive families.

Therefore, child welfare workers must work with a variety of family forms to produce successful outcomes for children and families. In the family-health perspective, family members define their family, which is an empowering process as long as the practitioner honors that definition (Pardeck & Yuen, 1997). Child-welfare practitioners who allow children and adolescents to describe their families will work with those persons, related or otherwise, who are significant to the children and who likely will be motivated to work for positive outcomes.

Because the family-health practice incorporates practice principles suggested by the systems, ecological, and strengths perspective, it is a good fit with foster-care services for families. For example, a worker using the systems theory considers how the family operates in relation to its broader environment; i.e., the practitioner considers what sources of stress and support flow into and out of the family to help it succeed, whether it is the biological, foster-care, or adoptive family. When a worker assesses child-abuse risk factors, s/he assesses the geographical and emotional isolation a family experiences, which explores the adaptations a family has made to and the niche it has carved for itself in its environment.

However, the traditional focus of practice with children in foster-care, has been deficit-based, highlighting the problems of families. And there are multiple problem areas that must be assessed in foster-care to produce safe and effective outcomes, including problems with early brain development, attachment to caregivers, sense of time and response to stress (Miller, Gorski, Borchers, Jenista, Johnson, Kaufman, Levitzky, Palmer & Poole, 2000). To be effective, services that are family-centered require strength-based strategies, which is a central feature of the family-health perspective (Jennings & Skibinski, 1997).

The strengths perspective directs professionals to not only find and utilize the strengths of families in foster-care but also to help families discover their own abilities and resources.. Strategies based on unique family strengths lead to innovative techniques, some of which are discussed in a later section of this chapter.

Foster-care services already employ interventions based on a strengths perspective. For example, many services to families now assess protective as well as risk factors. Protective factors include characteristics and resources of the child and family; e.g., perhaps the family has strong ties to a faith community that provides support and resources to family members or perhaps a child is an exceptional reader, which brings the child outside attention and encouragement.

Two practice principles have emerged in recent years to help the family discover its strengths. *Empowerment* is a process by which the family discovers its own strengths, while *resiliency* is the ability to use those strengths to its benefit (Corcoran & Nichols-Casebolt, 2004, Munroe, 2001). Using practice-principles interventions that enhance the resiliency and sense of empowerment of children, adolescents, and families can improve foster-care transitions and outcomes for biological families, kinship care families, foster families, and adoptive families.

Family-Health Principles for Empowerment in Foster Care

Empowerment in foster-care services begins with understanding the child's, adolescent's and family's construction of their reality, a key element of the family helath perspective. Clients must discover empowerment; it is not given to them by professionals (Payne, 2004). Strategies employed to discover the perspective of children and families address their need to feel more control over their placements and their lives (Johnson & Yoken, 1995; Munroe, 2001).

However, there has been little analysis of family perspectives on foster-care (Lindsey, 2001; Orme, 2001). It is rare to hear the view of the child. There is widespread agreement that children and adolescents have valuable perspectives on child welfare interventions, foster-care in particular (Festinger, 1983; Johnson & Yoken, 1995; Smith, 1996; Berrick, Frasch, & Fox, 2000; Kaplan, 2000). By seeking the views of children and families, a family-health practitioner promotes their empowerment.

One way to ascertain the perceptions of children and adolescents is to conduct a comprehensive assessment, which is a cornerstone of family-health practice. Bio-psycho-social assessments that address the physical, social, economic, cultural, emotional, spiritual, and mental domains of a family's life, are essential to discover problems and strengths common in foster-care situations (e.g., financial stress, support from cultural institutions). Such assessments should include the child's perspective as well as the perspective of every member of the family, avoiding the temptation to interview only the caregiver most available.

Comprehensive assessments include not only the development of the child, but that of the family as well. Age-appropriate intervention techniques rely on an assessment strategy sensitive to a child's development. Likewise, successful family assessments and interventions must consider family life cycles and family development. The use of genograms as a technique for assisting with such an assessment is discussed in a following section.

As part of a comprehensive assessment, foster-care workers must consider the external and internal stress a family is experiencing, a core principle of Minuchin's model of family therapy and the family-health perspective (Pardeck, 2002). The assessment not only identifies the stress a family experiences but also discovers the family's coping mechanisms because families are a powerful resource influencing the social functioning of individuals as well as larger systems (Pardeck, 2002).

In the family-health perspective, it is likewise essential to engage a family in an assessment of its cultural traditions, beliefs, and practices. For example, a family's culture will define stress and their reaction to stress. A worker's cultural competence moves beyond his/her understanding of a cultural group to one based on the family's definition of its culture. Strategizing for the family's cultural conceptualization of an issue is the most individualized source of empowerment for problem solving because it allows the family to identify their needs and strengths within their cultural context, which will drive how they respond and act.

Utilizing the support strategy of the family-health perspective is another way to empower families in the assessment process by discovering each member's view and construction of reality. While it involves time and the family context, the support strategy considers the child's view first, preventing other family members from defining an issue exclusively. Family members often need support to see the view of the child. The support strategy assists the family to discover what roles the child believes the family defined for each member. For example, a mother may say her child is depressed over a recent family break-up, while the child may say she is relieved over the dissolution but did not display such relief in deference to her mother. The child's view of herself and/or the issue should be as important, if not more so, than the mother's. In fact, the child may have a more accurate view of the issue.

Empowering children and families occurs in other stages of the helping process as well. For example, children can be empowered to participate meaningfully in the case- planning process. When given the opportunity, children in care request assistance to maintain relationships with biological families and foster families. Children request stability in families, friends, childcare and schools. Privacy and control are concerns of children and adolescents (Johnson & Yoken, 1995; Munroe, 2001; Thomas, N & O'Kane, 1999). However, if practitioners never seek the views of children and adolescents, the workers will never know what is significant to those groups.

Despite the strategy employed to empower children and adolescents in the foster-care system, it remains essential that foster-care practitioners develop relationships with children and adolescents through which children can explore what is happening in their families. Such relationships take time for numerous reasons (e.g., because children in foster care often do not trust authority figures) – time that is difficult to allow while respecting the children's pressing need to establish stability while in foster care. The family-health support strategy organizes assessment and intervention to prioritize time for the children to self-define in the family context. It is also important to remember that additional time is needed for termination of services with children in child welfare systems because it is a much slower process (Aiello, 1999).

Developing productive working relationships with children and families is the primary vehicle through which the practitioner creates an environment in which family members take the leading role in foster-care assessment, intervention, and termination. The family-health perspective draws attention to the family's role as the active director of activities that promote healthy lives and balances (Pardeck & Yuen, 2001). If children, adolescents, and families are active participants in foster-care services, they will discover their own sense of empowerment. Therefore, while children and families in the child welfare system are vulnerable they can be empowered with a combination of sensitive casework and encouragement to know their rights (Thomas and O'Kane, 1999).

Family-Health Practice Techniques for Empowerment in Foster Care

Family-health-practice strategies can enhance foster-care services by empowering children, adolescents, and families to take more control of their lives and a more active role in the child welfare processes. A basic principle of the family-health and strengths models is the individualization of any strategies to the needs and world view of the family members, so it is essential that practitioners solicit the family's perceptions of issues, needs, strengths, and plans. Following are examples of family-health-practice techniques effective in or adapted for use in foster-care services.

Genograms

From a family-health perspective, the use of genograms can assist with a developmental family assessment (e.g. foster family or family of origin) as well as with supportive and confrontive interventions. Genograms help the worker to recognize the level of prevention and readiness for change within the family. Further, genograms help utilize the family unit as a change agent and aid in understanding and assessing the construction of a child's reality (Pardeck et al., 1998).

Traditionally, child-welfare workers have used genograms mainly in adoption planning with foster parents (Pinderhughes & Rosenberg, 1990; Young, Corcoran-Rumpee, & Groze, 1992). However, genograms may be used for a variety of purposes in working with children involved in the foster-care system and be adapted age appropriately for individual clients. The worker can learn about the relations within the family of origin and the relationships with foster parents or kinship caregivers from the child's perspective (Altshuler, 1999). Involving the children in the construction of the genogram can promote engagement and as a tool to improve rapport. One way this is accomplished is by communicating to the children that the worker wants to get to know the family. The use of color markers helps engage the children in the genogram construction (Altshuler, 1999).

Genograms offer workers a better opportunity to grasp issues of cultural and/or ethnic differences between the worker and the children (Altshuler, 1999). Assisting with permanency planning from very early in the assessment process is another benefit of using genograms. Perhaps the greatest benefit of all is that the children are empowered by being actively involved as a member of the family. The entire family can also be empowered. Genograms can provide an accepted way of helping the worker, children and their family, whether it is a biological, foster, adoptive and/or kinship placement, achieve planning for the future (Altshuler, 1999).

Bibliotherapy

Most foster-care workers are familiar with bibliotherapy, the use of selected stories to facilitate discussion. A family-health practice technique would be to start with the family for ideas on themes. Allowing the family to choose the theme empowers them to guide the symbolism. An example would be selecting a story about an animal in need and an animal family that offers a home while searching for a parent. Or it could be the story of a boy who has magical powers who finds himself in a non-magical family that does not understand him. Families may relate to visual communication media as well as stories from books. The practitioner would ask the family for movies or television characters that they think illustrate their own positions and objectives.

Confrontive techniques

Direct confrontive techniques are more appropriate than interpretation when a child welfare worker is addressing childhood or youthful fantasies or idealizations. Adolescents particularly can hold on to identification with fantasized parents (Holman, 2001). Children and Adolescent may displace rage onto adoptive parents. Adoptive parents may have a hard time with the children's perspective if they are struggling with their own fear of abandonment. Appropriate confrontation may assist with mourning of parents as real people rather than idealized, tragic figures (Holman, 2001). Using the family-health perspective, a practitioner would first hear and understand the children's fantasies and would support them throughout the direct confrontation of the idealization. The worker would identify strengths the children have to overcome the loss of their fantasy and assist them is using such resources to grow and develop.

Visitation

Hess and Proch (1993) list the purposes of visiting: maintaining family relationships, coping with changing relationships, empowering and informing parents, enhancing children's well-being, helping families confront reality, providing a time and place to practice new behaviors, promoting accurate assessment, and providing a transition to home. Because of these goals, face-to-face visiting with biological parents is an intervention in most foster-care service plans but is greatly underutilized as a technique. Visits with the biological family can benefit the entire foster-care team, as well as empower children and families. Family-health-visiting techniques use clearly established goals and activities for the visits, which are based on the family's ideas for the shared time. In addition, practitioners are actively working with family members before, during, and after the visit to facilitate goals and to empower families to control the time they have together.

Narrative Therapy

Another adapted family-health technique that workers can utilize with age-appropriate foster-care children and families is narrative therapy or storytelling. Narrative therapy seeks the family's subjective view and focuses on empowerment. One aspect of storytelling helps the clients focus on incorporating an optimal worldview (Kirven, 2000). The technique would be useful in gathering information for a cultural assessment as families are allowed to tell their story from their own perspective.

Further, narrative therapy can address the spiritual domain of a family's life by incorporating a five-step strategy called Holistic Integration Techniques or H.I.T, which assists the clients to find meaning and build a spiritual connectedness to a higher power (Kirven, 2000). H.I.T. accomplishes this connection by helping children and families reframe hardships into constructive outcomes despite challenging conditions. H.I.T. also helps clients recognize strengths as well as limitations. Implementing better methods of functioning and coping within families' environments and working toward a more holistic way of functioning is an aim of H.I.T. These adapted family-health strategies empower children, adolescents, and families by allowing them to find and express their own voice, helping them to identify and use their strengths and allowing them to fail and succeed in a safe environment.

Candle Ceremony for Families

Family-health practice recognizes a variety of family forms. In foster-care, the family for intervention may not be the immediate living arrangement. There may be a need to "summarize" families in the past as a child moves to a different family. Candles are widely used in therapeutic settings as a means to help clients remember and move on. The candle ceremony in family-health practice is simple but empowering.

The family lights three candles, perhaps of different sizes or colors. One is for families in the past, one for the present family (including special mention of the child), and one for families in the future. Prior to the ceremony the family has listed particular strengths or remembrances of the child and families that they want to share with the lighting of each candle. The child keeps the candles for any desired future ceremonies.

Evaluation

Family-health practice utilizes evaluation as a technique in empowering families to impact systems at every level. On the individual level, evaluation can be used to confront family members. For example, contrasts could be spotlighted in family members' ratings after they use a scale to evaluate each others cooperativeness, or the family could evaluate the contributions they are currently making to development of a child.

Another useful evaluation technique is for children to describe on paper how others view them; the worker would then, with the child's permission, show parents their children's perceptions. Parents are sometimes surprised at the way children believe they are viewed. A parent that thought the child was fragile may find the child believes he/she is viewed as strong and resilient.

Evaluation as a group can be helpful for families in foster care. One subsystem that is often overlooked is biological siblings in a family providing care. Family Health Group sessions for these children can be the catalyst for their evaluations of benefits and challenges of being a foster family.

At the agency level empowerment in foster-care families might be evaluated with instruments such as the Family Hardiness Index (McCubbin, McCubbin & Thompson, 2000). The Hardiness Index measures a family's belief about controlling their experience and their commitment to and view of change. In foster-care, measures of hardiness appear to be specifically related to the intent of the substitute care family to continue fostering (Hendrix & Ford, 2003).

Family-health practitioners have a responsibility to evaluate a community's understanding and empowerment of foster-care families. Media coverage of family tragedies sways the public opinion of foster-care to extremes. Evaluation of the foster-care services in family-health practice involves rigorous but sensitive evaluation with the awareness that children label themselves when the community says foster care is "broken" or damaged beyond repair.

Record Keeping Techniques

Explaining client rights and obtaining informed consent are part of every entry into services. A remarkable empowerment occurs when children understand and are invited to sign the documents,for it gives them a sense of control over their experiences. In some situation a special document may be constructed not for legal purposes but for ethical ones, documenting children's rights, which further empowers them.

Adoption workers are familiar with the summaries that comprise the family history of children in care. A family-health-practice technique is to include sections of strengths and cultural traditions, with a broad definition of tradition. At some time in the future, these children will want to know about themselves and their heritage as part of a family of origin. Family-health practitioners would also allow children, adolescents, and families to contribute to their family history and records.

Care-plan meetings have been greatly improved with family-centered services and strength identification. There is a difference of opinion among members of care-plan teams regarding the participation of children in the planning meetings. Workers tend to believe the children should be present even if they are unable to fully understand the decisions of the group, while other professionals believe children should be excluded if they are not able to actively participate in the discussions (Shemmings, 2000). A family-health technique is to at least share a photo of the child as the plan is drafted. The child's image empowers the team to see the child as part of a family and not a conduit for their opinions on foster care. A family-health practitioner would meaningfully include children and adolescents in any case planning as often as possible.

Conclusion

In conclusion, our expectations of children and families in child-welfare systems have been focused through the lens of traditional medical and developmental models. Although these models have been helpful, they are limiting. Traditional models have been deficit-based, highlighting the expectation that children and families in child welfare systems will be at risk for health, education and mental health problems. If we expect children and families to be active, productive participants in the child-welfare system, we can help them discover empowerment and resilience through the use of family-health principles and suggested family-health techniques. These principles give preeminence to families' stories and view; give them active, meaningful roles in the assessment, intervention and termination processes; and recognize them as the directors of their helping processes. It is apparent that by themselves, child-welfare practitioners cannot solve families' problems; such resolution requires the empowerment and active involvement of children, adolescents, and families in the directions their lives take.

References

Aiello, T. (1999). *Child and adolescent treatment for social work practice: A Relational perspective for beginning clinicians*. New York: The Free Press.

Altshuler, S.J. (1999). Constructing genograms with children in care: Implications for casework practice. *Child Welfare, 78*, 777-790.

Berrick Duerr, J., Frasch, K., & Fox, A. (2000). Assessing children's experiences of out-of home care: Methodological challenges and opportunities. *Social Work Research, 24*,119-128.

Corcoran, J., & Nichols-Casebolt, A. (2004). Risk and resilience ecological framework for assessment and goal formulation. *Child and Adolescent Social Work Journal, 21*, 211-235.

Festinger, T. (1983). *No one ever asked us: A postscript to foster-care*. New York: Columbia University Press.

Hendrix, S., & Ford, J. (2003). Hardiness of foster families and the intent to continue to foster. *Journal of Family Social Work, 7*, 25-34.

Hess. P., & Proch, K. (1993). Visiting: The heart of reunification. In B.A. Pine, R. Warsh, & A.N. Maluccio. (Eds.), *Together again: Family reunification in foster-care*. Washington, DC: Child Welfare League.

Holman, W.D. (2001). Reaching for integrity: An Eriksonian life-cycle perspective on the experience of adolescents being raised by grandparents. *Child and Adolescent Social Work Journal, 18*, 21-34.

Jennings, M.A., & Skibinski, G.J. (1999). Treating families through a family-health perspective. In J.T. Pardeck & F.K.O. Yuen (Eds.), *Family-health: A holistic approach to social work practice* (pp. 45-59). Westport, CT: Auburn House.

Johnson, P.R., & Yoken, C. (1995). Family foster-care placement: The child's perspective. *Child Welfare, 74*, 959-975.

Kaplan, K.L. (2000). Young maltreated children's perceptions of their placement experiences. *Dissertation Abstracts International, 61* (7-A), 2593.

Kirven, J. (2000). Building on strengths of minority adolescents in foster-care: A narrative-holistic approach. *Child and Youth Care Forum, 29,* 247-263.

Lindsey, E.W. (2001). Foster family characteristics and behavioral and emotional problems of foster children: Practice implications for child welfare, family life education and marriage and family therapy. *Family Relations, 50,* 19-23.

McCubbin, M.A., McCubbin, H.I., & Thompson, A.I. (2000). Family hardiness index. In K. Corcoran & J. Fischer (Eds.). *Measures for clinical practice: A sourcebook* (3rd ed). New York: Free Press.

Miller, P.M., Gorski, P.A., Borchers, D.A., Jenista, J.A., Johnson, C.D., Kaufman, N.D., Levitzky, S.E., Palmer S.D., & Poole, J.M. (2000). Developmental issues for young children in foster-care. *Pediatrics, 106,* 1145-1151.

Munroe, E. (2001). Empowering looked-after children. *Child and Family Social Work, 6,* 129-137.

Orme, J.G. (2001). Foster family characteristics and behavioral and emotional problems of foster children: A narrative review. *Family Relations, 50,* 3-15.

Pardeck, J.T. (2002). Treating family stress through the family-health approach. In J.T. Pardeck (Ed.), *Family-health social work practice: A macro level approach* (pp. 57-70). Westport, CT.: Auburn House.

Pardeck, J.T., & Yuen, F.Y.O. (2001). Family-health: An emerging paradigm for social workers. *Journal of Health & Social Policy, 13,* 59-74.

Pardeck, J.T., & Yuen, F.K.O. (1997). A family-health approach to social work practice. *Family Therapy, 24,* 115-128.

Pardeck, J.T., Yuen, F.Y.O., Daley, J.G., & Hawkins, C. (1998). Social work assessment and intervention through family-health practice. *Family Therapy, 25,* 25-39.

Payne, M. (2004) *Modern social work theory*. Chicago: Lyceum Books, Inc.

Pinderhughes, E.E., & Rosenburg, K. (1990). Family-bonding with high-risk placements: A therapy model that promotes the process of becoming a family. In L.M. Glidden (Ed.), *Informed families: Adoption of children with handicaps.* New York: Haworth Press.

Shemmings, D. (2000). Professionals' attitudes to children's participation in decision-making: Dichotomous accounts and doctrinal contests. *Child and Family Social Work, 5,* 235-243.

Thomas, N., & O'Kane, C. (1999). Children's participation in reviews and planning meetings when they are 'looked-after' in middle childhood. *Child and Family Social Work, 4,* 221-230.

Chapter 14
Keeping Families Together by Promoting Family Health
Frank G. Kauffman

The focus of this chapter is on the impact of intensive family preservation services (IFPS) on the holistic well-being of families with children who are at risk for abuse and neglect. The principal underlying goal of family preservation and family support programs is to decrease the placement of children in foster care and other residential settings by providing in-the-home services to parents and caregivers. Family preservation programs embrace a "nonjudgmental" ethic of providing services to *all* families no matter how dysfunctional and abusive.

The family health perspective holds that the goal of the family unit is to develop and maintain a healthy interaction among seven domains that directly impact the well-being and functioning of its members (Pardeck & Yuen 1999). This perspective has its origins in systems theory. According to Bowen (1990) this theory holds that the family unit is a naturally occurring system that exhibits patterns of emotional functioning (instinctual rather than feeling) and that therapeutic interventions directed to any member of the unit can modify or change the behavior of all members of the unit. Given this framework, family health is "a state of holistic well-being of the family system" (Pardeck & Yuen 1999, p. 1).

The chapter will also discuss the relationship of family preservation services to family health, the characteristics of parents and children in abusive families, the role of social workers, and implications for family-health practitioners.

Family Health vs. Family Preservation

The family-health perspective is a relatively new approach utilized to assess and guide the treatment interventions of family dysfunction from a systems perspective. The family is viewed as the source from which most problems exist. The model is based on four key concepts as articulated by Pardeck and Yuen (1997). The first emphasizes the client family as the source for their beliefs about health and behavior. The work of Minuchin (1974) and Pratt (1976) reinforces the relationship between family illness and how the family functions as a unit within the context of their environment and culture. Behaviors may be both positive (as in diet and exercise) and negative or harmful (as in smoking, substance abuse, violence, or homelessness or isolation).

The second concept is the role of stress as it impacts family health and functioning. A number of studies suggest that stress represents a direct correlation with certain types of disease including heart disease, hypertension, and obesity. Stress is also correlated with poverty, unemployment, underemployment, and social isolation.

Third, in order for practitioners to be effective in the assessment and intervention of family dysfunction, they must understand that client families may not be able to break or change the patterns of dysfunctional behavior. A level of dysfunction is essential for maintaining some sort of homeostasis. It may require the learning and implementing of new behaviors that may be uncomfortable or foreign to those families.

Finally, the worker must focus on the family as the source of strength and courage with which to change patterns of behavior and thus improve family functioning. In doing so the worker emphasizes family strengths as a source for understanding and changing dysfunctional behaviors.

Family preservation programs were designed to keep families together and improve family functioning. Although the underlying goal was to keep families together by reducing the risk for abuse and neglect of children, its overall goal is

216

to improve family functioning by teaching and modeling new behaviors for family members. Programs share a "common philosophy of family centered services including focusing on family strengths, involving families in determining their treatment plans including goals, serving the entire family, and treating families with respect" (Schuerman & Rossi, 1995, p.3).

Most family-preservation programs are predicated on crisis intervention theory. According to Caplan (1964) a crisis is defined as an "upset in a steady state that poses and obstacle, usually important to the fulfillment of important life goals or to vital need satisfaction, and that the individual or family cannot overcome through usual methods of problem solving" (p. 418). Further, Hepworth & Larson (1993) suggest that during a period of crisis the individual or family is presented the option of doing something positive to overcome the crisis or something destructive that aggravates the crisis. Thus, family-preservation programs are designed to assist the family in making the best decision that will overcome the crisis and assist the family in regaining some degree of pre-crisis functioning.

The family health perspective and family preservation both imply/suggest that improved family functioning as well as the holistic well-being of families is contingent on their relationship and interaction with the larger environment in which they exist.

Family-Preservation Services Improving Family Health

Family preservation services are provided in the home with the goal of working with the family as a system. Under systems theory positive outcomes including improvement in family functioning can occur from two perspectives: 1) the theory that change in the individual will lead to changes in the family unit, or 2) change in the group leads to change within the individual. Either perspective embraces a "nonjudgmental" ethic of providing services to all families no matter how dysfunctional or abusive.

The concept of in-the-home services to families stems from the Elizabethan Poor Laws of the 17th century when "outdoor" relief was replaced by "indoor" relief or institutional care (Morton and Grigsby, 1993). The laws represented the first time that state intervention would determine who was eligible for what services and how services would be provided.

In 1909 the White House Conference on Children emphasized a public commitment to assist children in their homes. This commitment was based on the value of "home life," the "highest and finest product of civilization, children should not be deprived of it except for urgent and compelling reasons" (Morton et al. 1993, p. 7). Subsequent legislation further supported the importance of keeping families together including the 1965 Aid to Families with Dependent Children (AFDC). This piece of legislation supported and reinforced the premise that family and home life was essential for maintaining the holistic well-being of families.

Family-preservation services are provided based on two entirely different models. One, the Homebuilder's model, emphasizes the intensive, short-term nature of providing services for periods of four to six weeks working with the family approximately ten or more hours per week. The other, considered a traditional model, suggests that services be provided over longer periods of time, anywhere from 90 to 160 days with the average at 120 days. The actual time spent with the family is about three to six hours per week, depending on the severity of the situation or degree of dysfunction. The success or failure of these two models is measured in "placement prevention rates" or PPR. Although PPR are not the focus of this examination, suffice it to say that both models are considered effective in keeping families together and maintaining the holistic well-being and thereby reducing placement prevention rates.

According to the Annie E. Casey Foundation (1999) there are six primary risk factors that impact family well-being and the future outcomes of children. Those factors and the percentage of at-risk children experiencing them are as follows:

Single parent (s)	32%
Parent or caregiver is a high school dropout	19%
Family income is below the poverty line	21%

Under or unemployment of parent or care giver	28%
Family is on welfare	12%
Children without health insurance	15%

These coupled with other risk factors such as drug/substance abuse, domestic violence, family isolation, and mental illness, the chances of having a child placed outside the home increase exponentially.

The number of risk factors experienced by a family is directly correlated with higher placement rates of children (Schorr, 1991; Pecora, 1991; Magura, 1981; and Jones, 1985). Dr. Lisbeth Schorr (1991) argues that the more risk factors experienced by a family, the "greater damaging impact of each." She also states that the impact of each factor is not necessarily additive; rather, "risk factors multiply each other's destructive effects (p. 261)."

Characteristics of the parent/caregiver and children at risk for abuse and neglect can be as comprehensive as to include every situation or, as outlined by Kauffman (2002), may be reduced to the following characteristics: parents or caregivers usually prefer corporal punishment when disciplining their children; verbal discipline, when used, is often negative and hostile; failure to assume the parental role; are not affectionate or approving and, in fact, may openly reject the child; and prefers or may request an out-of-home placement for the child.

The characteristics of children may include, but are not limited to, poor school attendance, delinquent behavior including property crimes or crimes against others, involvement in drugs or alcohol, or self destructive behavior.

The risk factors coupled with the characteristics of abusive parents and their children require that a comprehensive assessment and treatment plan be developed that meets the needs of families and contributes to their holistic well-being.

Assessment, Treatment, and Intervention

As a model for assessment and intervention the family-health perspective provides the worker with a comprehensive view of the areas or domains that impact family functioning and well-being. For example, a referral from a state agency substantiating abuse and neglect typically reports on the relevant issues surrounding the allegations of abuse or neglect. It does not take into account other, relevant variables that may or may not be a contributing factor in placing children at risk for abuse and neglect.

The basic premises of the family-health perspective (Pardeck & Yuen, 1997) compare favorably with the goals of family preservation interventions in producing positive outcomes for families. Family health has its foundations in a psychosocial orientation that places family problems in a larger social context. Therefore at-risk families are viewed as part of a larger social system. Second, family health practice views the family as the fundamental unit of analysis. The family is the expert in defining their beliefs regarding health and health seeking behavior. Third, family health oriented workers value the collaborative efforts of other professionals when working with client families. The family preservation worker may, in fact, rely on linking other professionals with the client family.

Finally, family health practitioners providing services to at-risk families view themselves as being, "in" or "apart of" rather than being separate from the family during the intervention. The worker is able to model appropriate behaviors and is able to work with the families as they begin to implement those new behaviors.

These concepts or premises are important in light of the range of treatment outcomes reported in the literature (Kinney, Haapala and Booth 1991, Berry 1992, Rossi 1991, 1992, and Pecora 1991). According to these studies placement prevention rates have ranged from 60 to 90% during and following treatment. Two of the most often cited studies (Feldman 1991, Schuerman, Rzepknicki, and Littell 1994) found no statistical relationship between implementation of family preservation services and placement prevention rates. Schuerman's study noted that placement prevention rates in the experimental group were higher than in the treatment group.

The majority of the studies conducted on the effectiveness of family preservation programs in reducing placement prevention rates have used some sort of control group, primarily "overflow" groups of client families who could not receive services or be assigned to treatment groups. This raised ethical questions regarding informed consent, random selection, and additional questions regarding the heterogeneity of the client families.

In order to develop a comprehensive intervention the worker must consider the physical, mental, emotional, social, economic, cultural, and spiritual dimensions that correlate with family functioning and positive outcomes for client families. The importance of the treatment plan cannot be overstated. According to Pecora (1991) an effective treatment plan is instrumental in improving family functioning, leading to successful outcomes. In families with children at risk for abuse and neglect, the children of families who met most or all of the treatment goals were more likely to remain in the home. In fact, the risk of treatment failure was approximately 64% lower than in those families who failed to meet their treatment goals. The treatment plan, developed with input from the client family, identifies goals and objectives to be accomplished during the treatment period.

Implications for Family Health Practitioners

Social workers providing services to families with children at risk for abuse and neglect working from the family-health perspective are prepared to assess not only biological and social factors attendant in client families but also factors from the "person, family, community, and the social context of the person-in-the environment" (Pardeck & Yuen, 1997, pp. 125 to 126). In other words, the worker will consider *all* aspects and interactions of the client family and their relationship with the larger social environment. Although poverty is directly correlated with child abuse and neglect, other factors also contribute to the problem and beg for attention. For example, a worker providing services to a family considered middle-upper or upper class may not be aware of risk factors not facing lower-middle class families or those living in poverty with its attendant problems and risk factors. Although the risk factors and presenting problems may be devastating to the holistic well-being of the family of either socio-economic class, the worker will benefit by an awareness of the dimensions or domains that may represent risks to the client family. In his or her assessment the worker will have an advantage in understanding the various dimensions that contribute to or detract from family functioning. Other assessment tools including genograms and ecomaps are useful in diagramming in order to gain a comprehensive assessment of the source of the family's dysfunction and other related or environmental factors that place children at risk for abuse and neglect.

Conclusion

The family-health perspective provides the worker with a model or discipline with which to work with families with children who are at risk for abuse and neglect. When the worker is able to assess the domains or dimensions that impact family functioning and well-being, the potential for successful outcomes is enhanced. The family health perspective allows the worker to move beyond the family as the primary source of dysfunction and focus on how the family functions and interacts with the environment in which they exist and interact. The family is looked on as not functioning in a vacuum unaffected by their environment. This is not to say that the family wouldn't be the source of the dysfunction; rather, it expands the worker's knowledge and effectiveness when assessing and working with families with children at risk for abuse and neglect.

References

Berry, M. (1992). "An evaluation of family preservation services: Fitting agency services to family needs." *Social Work, 37*(4), 314-321.

Caplan. G. (1964). *Principles of preventive psychiatry.* New York: Basic Gook, Inc.

Feldman, L. H. (1991). "Assessing the effectiveness of family preservation services in New Jersey within an ecological context." New Jersey Division of Youth and Family Services, Bureau of Research, Evaluation, and Quality Assurance, Trenton, NJ.

Hepworth, D. H. and Larsen, J. (1993). *Direct social work practice: Theory and skills.* Pacific Grove, CA: Brooks/Cole.

Kauffman, F. G. (2002). *Preventing child abuse and neglect in Arizona: Perceptions of the homebuilders' model.* Unpublished doctoral dissertation, Arizona State University.

Kinney, J., Haapala, D., & Booth, C. (1991). *Keeping families together: The homebuilders' model.* New York: Aldine De Gruyter.

Jones, M. (1985). A *second chance for families: Five years later.* New York: Child Welfare League of America.

Magura, S. (1981). "Are services to prevent foster care effective?" *Children and Youth Services Review, 3,* 193-212.

Morton, G. and Grigsby, R. (Eds). (1993*). Advancing family preservation practice.* Newbury Park, CA: Sage Publications

Minuchin, S. (1974). *Families and family therapy.* Cambridge, MA: Harvard University Press

Pardeck, J. & Yuen, F. K. (1999). *Family health: A holistic approach to social work practice.* Westport, CT: Auburn House.

Pecora, P. J. (1991). "Family-based and intensive family preservation services: A select literature review." In Fraser. M., Pecora, J. & Haapala, D. (Eds), *Families in crisis: The impact of intensive family preservation services.* New York: Aldine De Gruyter.

Pratt, L. (1976). *Family structure and effective health behavior: The energized family.* Boston: Houghton-Mifflin.

Rossi, P. H. (1992). "Assessing family preservation programs." *Children and Youth Services Review, 14,* 77-97.

Schorr, L. (1991). *Effective programs for children growing up in concentrated poverty.* In Huston, A. C., (Ed.) *Children in poverty.* University of Cambridge Press, p. 261-262.

Schuerman, J. & Rossi, P. (1995). *A review of family preservation and family reunification programs.* The Chapin Hall Center for Children at the University of Chicago. Retrieved July 26, 2004, from http://aspe.hhs.gov/cyp/fpprogs.htm.

Schuerman, J. Rzepknicki, T., & Littell, J. (1994). *Putting families first: An experiment in family preservation.* New York: Aldine De Gruyter.

STUDIES IN HEALTH AND HUMAN SERVICES